GET IT STRAIGHT

YOUNG, SEXY
AND HEALTHY!

Dr. Elma Schnapp, M.D.
& Dr. Moacir Schnapp, M.D.

©2007 Dr. Elma Schnapp and Dr. Moacir Schnapp
Photographs: Beto Riginik
LifeART images © 2007 Lippincott Williams & Wilkins. All rights reserved.

Design and lay out: Disciple Design

Published by Colletes and Sons

Schnapp, Elma and Schnapp, Moacir
        Young, Sexy and Healthy: The Ten Best Exercises for Your Posture.

ISBN-13 978-0-9719337-4-3 paperback
ISBN-10 0-9719337-4-X paperback

Visit our website
iposture.com

Contents

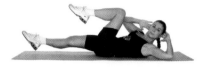

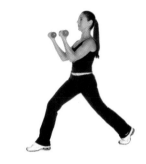

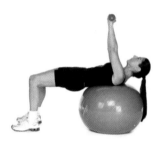

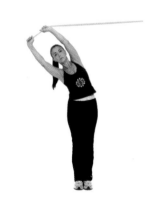

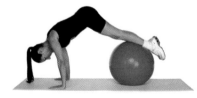

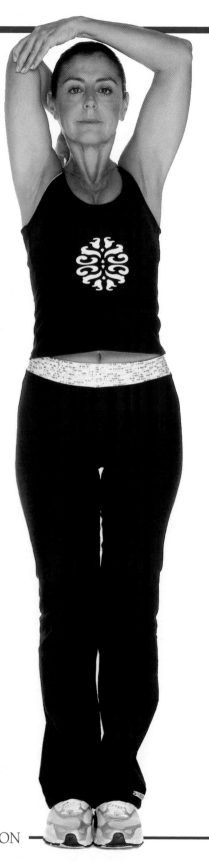

Introduction

Why another fitness book, you may ask? A trip to your local bookstore and a quick glance at the never-ending, ever-growing health section aisle will give you an idea of the huge number of publications available on fitness and exercise. It seems that everything that could be printed about keeping fit already has. It is also readily apparent that most of these books have been written by people who are passionate about their craft and about fitness in general, people who believe that they can contribute something to the health and well-being of others. And you know what? So do I.

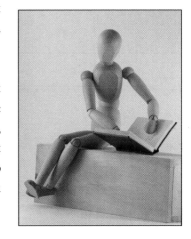

I belong to the majority of people who wish they were taller. As I get older my original height of 5'4" is no more; I have to look up to face my kids and I must tiptoe to reach the top shelves. I hate to admit it, but gravity is slowly taking a toll on my precious body. Still, I'm not going to give up without a fight, and I'm certainly "not going to go gentle into that good night." I refuse to give away any height that I can possibly manage to keep.

"Life is what happens while you're busy making plans," once said my favorite Beatle, John Lennon. Many moons ago, a career-ending knee injury derailed my plans to become a professional dancer, leaving me no other choice but to pursue my other passion, medicine. As a physician who has specialized in rehabilitation and as an avid exerciser, I've had the chance over many years to polish and refine a fitness program, which I hope I can pass on to our readers. I want to do so in a way that is fun and that reflects my joy for life and the respect that I have for that wonderful machine that is the human body. The routine of exercises that I offer the readers in this book is the same one that I have developed and perfected for myself and which I have practiced for years. It encompasses a combination of stretching, weight training, aerobic exercises, and postural workouts designed to maintain one's height, strength, and balance.

I have added some basic medical information, which I believe every person who exercises should have, written in terms that I hope will be easily understood. It is a challenge to avoid being too basic or too complex when describing and explaining things such as exercise physiology or the medical conditions that affect a fitness program. My apologies.

I hope the readers understand the extra space and special attention devoted in this book to the bone and muscle loss that affects individuals as they age; it is, after all, one of my main areas of interest and a major public health issue. I have also included medical prevention tips for our younger readers who could benefit from my experience, hoping that they may avoid some of the pitfalls incurred by their parents.

Even though it is my face you'll see on the exercises in this book, it is my husband, Dr. Moacir Schnapp, who is, for the most part, responsible for this manuscript, transforming my loose thoughts, concepts, and ideas into a comprehensible language, adding from his knowledge on the subject, and utilizing his expertise in communicating with his patients to make this what I hope will be an easy to understand and enjoyable book.

Being Tall is an Attitude

I don't get cramped in coach. I can buy at any department store's petite section. If I fall, it will be from a lesser height than taller people. I can easily enter even the smallest of sports cars, and I don't have to duck when boarding a helicopter. Nevertheless, society favors taller specimens, probably as a biological tool for the survival of the species. Good teeth, unblemished skin, and bright eyes, for example, are signs of beauty in most any culture. Height is another universal marker for beauty and health, but regrettably, for the rest of us, a couple of inches of added height frequently translate into a fatter paycheck or a better shot at a promotion. It also means I'll never work as a showgirl in Vegas.

Then again, I believe that being tall is an attitude: not just feet and inches on a ruler, but a state of mind that reflects the way we feel about ourselves. Our posture, more than our physical height, dictates how happy or successful others perceive us to be. For instance, the slouching stance of a fast growing teenager, unaccustomed to the rapid changes in the muscles and bones that occur in adolescents, is often erroneously interpreted as a lack of confidence or self-esteem. On the other hand, the perfect posture of a diminutive female Olympic gymnast packed with powerful muscles is a compelling enough symbol of success to guarantee an endorsement to sell Wheaties.

Oddly enough, our body language, like the posture and the facial expressions we display every day, also have a profound influence on the way we think and act. The effect that our posture has on the way we behave is a well-known fact among psychology specialists but hidden from much of the general public.

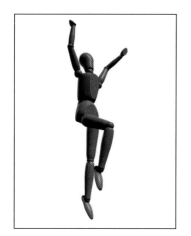

Our body language shapes how our brain thinks, how it reacts to common, everyday events and, ultimately, how the nervous system makes decisions. In a classic psychological study, a multiple-choice questionnaire designed to measure happiness and optimism was administered to a group of individuals. Half of them were instructed to maintain a smile on their face while answering the test questions while the other half were asked to keep frowning during the same experiment. When the answers were analyzed, it showed that the frowning group consistently showed a higher rate of pessimistic answers, denoting greater unhappiness than the smiling group even though both portrayed only a "fake" emotion.

Perhaps the human brain and that of other animals are already "hard-wired" for emotional reaction in response to our body language, as well as the reaction to the body language of our peers. For instance, primates such as monkeys are known to slouch or bow in order to avoid harassment and to escape harm by other members of their group. They often lower the body enough to lift their behind in the air as a sign of submission during a threatening encounter; the alpha male, on the other hand, shows off to his peers by assuming a typical, exaggerated, upright posture.

A friend of mine gave me this advice when I was looking for a job: "You should dress for the job you want, not for the job you have." To that, I would add: "...and you should display the posture for the person you want to be." Supermodels are not the only ones whose careers are affected by posture; all sorts of working people, from a saleswoman in Alabama to an attorney in Washington, anyone who deals with the public may enhance their professional standing by acquiring a posture that communicates empathy, confidence, and pride in the work they do. Just about every other book written about how to succeed in business mentions the proper stance, the right clothes, and the perfect handshake, as among the fundamental building blocks for one's career advancement. Remember that the posture you display not only communicates your level of confidence to others, but it also tunes your mind to positive, optimistic attitudes that reinforce the message that a successful person wants to convey.

A perfect posture doesn't come naturally for most of us, and I, for one, have to work hard at maintaining mine in the hope that the positive outcome to my body and my mind are worth the effort. Can I change my posture in a positive way that increases my comfort and health? Can my poise give me more confidence and add success to my career? Can my stance prevent my body from showing its age? If so, sign me up.

What is Good Posture?

Structures like bridges or skyscrapers sometimes behave in unpredictable ways, challenging the engineers who build them to forecast and prevent any possible catastrophic failure. They know that every building they design is more than the sum of its parts, and they must match the architecture of the building with its surroundings, allowing it to behave in harmony with itself and the environment. A classic example of what can go wrong when we ignore that 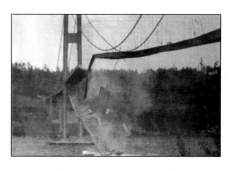 interaction was the destruction of the Tacoma Narrows Bridge in Washington, torn to pieces in 1940 by the strong winds that regularly blow in that area. The winds responsible for such damage were not very strong, but they were coincidentally tuned to the natural swaying frequency of that bridge, comparable to pushing a child on a swing higher and higher.

The human body is a machine far more complex than anything engineers could build, each one of us containing a distinctive combination of muscles, bones, and nerves that behave in a unique way, subjected to different forces and different environments. I picture the interaction of these multiple parts and the resulting motion that comes from it as a melody, the harmony that comes from playing just the right notes or from moving just the right muscles. It would be presumptuous for anybody to try to apply a cookie cutter model or a single formula to determine the perfect posture for everyone regardless of age, sex, or cultural background, for instance. Instead, I hope that by following the guidelines we set in this book, each one of you may come across your own personal, unique, feel-good stance. Once you discover your perfect, harmonious posture, you may find yourself more relaxed, confident, and energized. The combination of the correct posture and a faithful exercise program may reduce or eliminate a variety of aches and pains that affect us all, while decreasing the stiffness and fatigue that creep in as we age.

As difficult as it is to define, good standing posture certainly isn't the hard, inflexible soldier's stance: inflated chest, standing at attention. It is perhaps better defined as a posture that imparts a feeling of lightness: head reaching upwards like helium balloons attached to the top of one's skull. A person's correct stance has to feel comfortable, relaxing, and natural; it should merge seamlessly into one's personality and daily routine, as cozy as a favorite sweater.

There are many reasons why holding a proper posture may make us feel better:

· The right stance allows the bones and joints in the spinal column to remain aligned and balanced, avoiding the damage that arises from excessive straining.

· It creates an environment where the muscles of the trunk can operate at their maximum efficiency and with less wear, allowing them to relax when not in use and therefore minimizing fatigue.

· It reduces the occurrence of low back problems as well as the likelihood of developing the tense, painful neck and shoulders that plague so many of us at the end of a hard day.

Some fortunes you inherit; some you create. Certain people are lucky enough to be born with the right kind of genes that may afford them, for example, an impeccable set of teeth, a hawk-like vision, or even an effortless perfect posture. The rest of us, mere mortals, may need to wear braces, glasses, or we may need to work real hard for that awe-inspiring stance we covet. If we didn't inherit it, we'll have to get it the old-fashioned way: by exercising and modifying our lifestyle to overcome our genetic limitations.

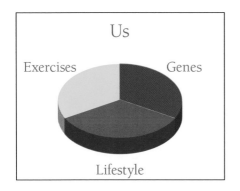

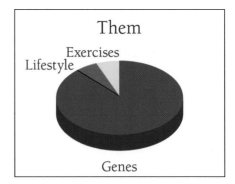

The Internal Organs and Posture

Breathing

The health benefits obtained by developing a proper stance are not restricted to the musculoskeletal system but extend to all areas of the body. For instance, the lungs can do their best job when our posture is good enough to allow the rib cage and the diaphragm muscle to expand properly. The exchange of oxygen between the lungs and the blood is thus improved, and less effort is required to breathe and speak.

It's easy to take breathing for granted, and we often forget that when inhaling we don't really pull any air in; instead, we just expand the thorax and the abdomen outwards so air rushes in passively to fill in the vacuum this expansion creates. Adequate posture is essential for proper breathing during all kinds of exercises, but it is particularly important during competitive sports because of the high oxygen demand (you never see sprinters slouching during the one hundred meter dash). Even less challenging activities, like singing, require a good posture. Any experienced voice coach will tell you that proper posture is a must for a singer's voice to sound strong, travel far, and do so without strain.

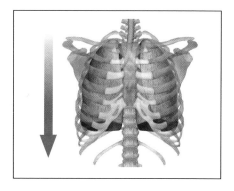

If you want further proof of the importance of one's stance when breathing, try this experiment: curl your spine and shoulders into a slouched position, exhale, and hold your breath. Now try to stand up straight while still holding your breath. You'll feel the vacuum that is created inside your chest and abdomen when you correct your posture, compelling you to take a breath. This represents the amount of breathing space you lose, the extra lung volume you're missing when you're slouched.

Digestion

When it comes to the digestive system, proper posture allows the internal organs in the abdomen to assume their natural position without undue compression, which can interfere with the normal flow and function of the gastrointestinal apparatus. An improper, slouched posture has been postulated as a contributing factor to several digestive problems, from acid reflux to constipation and even hernias.

Form follows function, and standing up straight not only allows the abdominal organs to function better, but it also improves the shape of the body in ways that are immediate and profound. For instance, one of the major complaints of mature women (and men) is a growing "belly pouch," an abdominal distention that afflicts even thin people as they age and that can't be resolved by liposuction or sit-ups alone because it is due to the protruding viscera pushing against the abdominal wall. The shrinking internal volume of the abdomen that forces the guts to bulge is mostly due to the loss of height of the lumbar spine that accompanies age (think of what happens when you squeeze an Oreo cookie). By straightening up the body, you can trim several inches from the waist simply by increasing the distance between your lower ribs and the pelvis, allowing greater volume for the internal organs to spread and instantaneously reducing an unsightly "beer belly" or a "grandmotherly bulge."

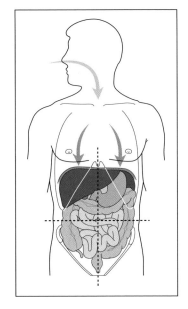

What Causes Poor Posture?

Growing Up

For generations, youngsters have had to endure a never-ending hassle about their posture from parents and well-wishing relatives. "Straighten up!" or "Don't slouch!" are still the mantra in many households.

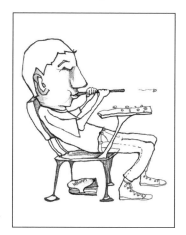

Teens frequently sabotage what would otherwise be a perfect posture for a variety of reasons, but we often find its origins linked to the rapid changes that normally occur to the bodies of adolescents. Boys may stoop to reduce their newfound height, or just to try to seem less conspicuous, while girls have been known to do the same to hide their budding breasts. Nowadays, other challenges for teens trying to keep their posture abound, including the extensive and intensive use of computers, video games, and the all-pervasive TV, all of which certainly don't help a youngster's stance. Some forms of self-expression teens adopt, like the dark, gothic, hunched-over persona displayed by a certain segment of the high school population, can certainly lead to poor posture.

Adulthood

Grown-ups have their own reasons to display poor posture, but fatigue is very likely one of the preponderant causes. Tension and tiredness develop quickly with such day-to-day stressors like work, kids, errands, and bills. Pretty soon the weight of the world rests on one's shoulders; it's no wonder we slump.

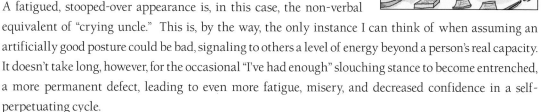

Psychologists may tell you that a less obvious reason adults slouch is that, unconsciously, we use it as a non-verbal means to communicate to our peers and family how we actually feel. We often assume this poor, hunched-over posture and body language as a warning to our colleagues, boss, or spouse that we already have enough work, chores, or responsibilities to do, and we should not be given any more tasks. A fatigued, stooped-over appearance is, in this case, the non-verbal equivalent of "crying uncle." This is, by the way, the only instance I can think of when assuming an artificially good posture could be bad, signaling to others a level of energy beyond a person's real capacity. It doesn't take long, however, for the occasional "I've had enough" slouching stance to become entrenched, a more permanent defect, leading to even more fatigue, misery, and decreased confidence in a self-perpetuating cycle.

In addition, the lack of a regimented exercise program is one of the main reasons for the poor posture many adults carry. While most teens can stay in shape without exercise, adults have a harder time keeping their muscle mass, a basic requirement to keep the spine straight. A fitness program becomes a more pressing necessity as we age, but most adults don't really follow one. Many of us, instead, choose to buy an expensive treadmill or a stationary bike, fooled into believing that if we spend enough money on state of the art exercise machines we'll feel too guilty not to use them; it seldom works, and the state of the art equipment often end up as very expensive clothes hangers.

"I'm too busy" is the most common excuse adults use to justify the lack of an adequate, solid exercise program when, in fact, a routine of exercises not only improves stamina but also our ability to focus and concentrate, which readily pays off in increased productivity at work and in one's life in general. Bottom line? More time and energy left at the end of the day.

Growing Old

This is when things get really complicated. Aging is one of those pre-programmed, built-in functions of every cell contained in the body. The fancy name for cell death is apoptosis, a phenomenon that occurs spontaneously after a cell divides and reproduces a certain number of times. The tips of the chromosomes, the elongated structures inside the nucleus of the cell that contain our body's genetic information, get shorter and shorter each time a cell divides, until it eventually can't divide anymore. This means that all the tissues that compose the body will eventually fail, including bones, joints, and muscles.

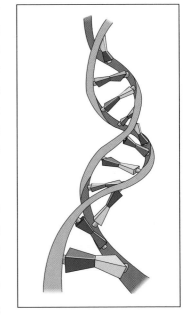

In the absence of a fountain of youth, people grasp at any new development, tenuous as it may be, to slow down this inexorable aging clock. Desperation turns otherwise smart individuals into easy prey for advertisements that sell anything that even remotely sounds like it could help them, ranging from vitamins and natural/organic foodstuffs to esoteric products that claim that something like "energized water" is the solution to all that ails us. Sadly, despite the devotion of a great many scientists and a sizeable amount of money spent on longevity research, the only proven method that allows an animal to live substantially longer requires a reduction in the number of calories ingested, an average of ten percent less than an animal's daily requirement. Laboratory rats subjected to this very low calorie diet may live twice as long as their counterparts fed regular meals. Scientists are still looking for proof that this diet of partial starvation could be effective and safe for humans. Before you decide to embark on such a regimen, remember that even moderate degrees of malnutrition can cause irreparable damage to the body, decreasing one's defenses against infections and slowing down the metabolism. Stay tuned for further developments.

We may not yet know the secret to longevity, but we do have some clues as to what can be done to improve our quality of life, especially on how to feel better through the second half of our lifespan. For starters, we must choose wisely among the myriad of medical and lifestyle options that present themselves to us, seeking only those that would be indeed relevant and meaningful to our health, selecting the ones most likely to benefit us (not an easy task to accomplish in a world of misinformation, media hype, and infomercials). The vast amounts of time, energy, and money spent on catchy but unproven health methods means that less is left to spend on tried and true techniques.

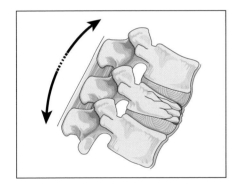

We tend to place our limited intellectual and financial resources on the wrong kind of problems. For instance, most people worry much more about flying and plane crashes (a relatively rare event), than driving and car accidents (a major, everyday source of disability and death). Beachgoers are more likely to watch out for sharks than riptides, even though the numbers of people who drown are many times higher than those who succumb to Jaws. Similarly, accidents and falls are among the most important preventable causes of disability, but they don't get much airtime on TV. One million osteoporosis fractures occur annually in the US, many times with life-changing consequences. Age leads to muscle atrophy, decreased balance and vision, impaired cardiovascular function, and loss of nerve cells, all contributing to decreased reflexes and consequently to the increased number of accidents observed in mature folks. Accident avoidance is more important for health maintenance than most medical interventions: wearing a seat belt is more likely to benefit us than drinking organic vegetable juices, and holding on to the hand-rail while going downstairs is more useful than an expensive air purifier.

One of the top accident prevention measures is the regular use of a fitness program, shown over and over again as among the best, most reliable approach to enhance one's balance and to reduce the number of accidental falls. Many physiologic explanations have been postulated to explain the benefits of this exercise-induced stability, including greater muscle mass and better heart and lung functions, but it seems that the central nervous system may be the greatest beneficiary from such a fitness program. It has been convincingly demonstrated that physical activity does improve and even creates connections between the nerve cells in the nervous system, an actual learning process that happens at a cellular level essentially no different from what occurs when one learns to play an instrument. In addition, it also enhances the blood flow to the brain and increases intellectual capacity. Even lab rats allowed to play and exercise are less likely than their counterparts to develop the so-called amyloid plaques in the brain, a hallmark of Alzheimer's disease. The result is that an exercise routine leads to quicker reflexes, better coordination, improved inner ear function, and decrease in the number of dizzy spells that plagues us as we age, therefore reducing the chances for accidents.

Osteoporosis

Osteoporosis deserves a special chapter in this book since it is by far the most important preventable cause of irreversible posture changes in adults. Osteoporosis is a progressive damage to the architecture of the bones, not to be confused with osteoarthritis, the natural wear and tear of the body joints that will eventually affect all of us. Instead, osteoporosis is related to a decrease in the calcium and the structural protein that maintains the bone's strength and flexibility; it may lead to a weakening of any and all of the bones in the body, but in a particularly vicious way, it affects the spine and the hips. Unchecked, osteoporosis may cause permanent anatomical changes in the spine, from micro fractures to full breaks that can cause a vertebrae to collapse with consequent loss of height and changes in the curvature of the spinal column. Misery loves company, and spinal fractures beget more spinal fractures due to the additional stress exerted by the abnormal curvature.

The long bones of the body, the feet, and the hands are also commonly affected, leading to other problems such as hip, wrist, and ankle breaks. Hip fractures that were once thought to be mostly the result of falls, are instead, many times the result of a spontaneous fracture that occurs while the person is just standing or walking, then followed by a fall, such is the degree of bone fragility developed in severe osteoporosis.

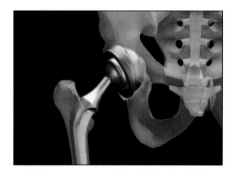

We often think about the bones as solid, immutable structures, whose only function is to sustain the rest of the body. Truth is, bones are made of live tissue that display a continuous turnover and are constantly being remade, same as the skin and other tissues. The skeleton is a repository for calcium, a buffer that limits what could be dangerous calcium fluctuations in our system, lending some calcium to the blood when it is needed only to acquire it back at the first chance. As we get older this process is subverted, and calcium deposition begins to lag the calcium that leaves the bone with a resultant net skeletal loss. To some extent, this loss is inevitable and progressive, and the best we can do is to fight to slow it down.

Osteoporosis in its early stages is a painless ailment, and it may remain undiagnosed for many years, delaying proper treatment until the weakened bones do fail and break. Insidious at first, one may initially notice only some loss of height and changes in the curve of the spine; the first sign of a real problem for the majority of people is an acute fracture.

Early detection and therapy of osteoporosis is the only way to slow down the bone loss to prevent skeletal deformities. For a proper diagnosis of osteoporosis, the density of the bone should be determined through the use of specialized X-rays. Although bone density is the most commonly utilized method to detect and quantify osteoporosis, it does not reveal the specific causes for the bone loss; those may include varied medical conditions like kidney diseases, parathyroid gland abnormalities, and even malabsorption due to intestinal problems such as Crohn's disease.

Although calcium gets most of the attention when it comes to the health and integrity of the bones, truth is that the protein matrix that makes up the skeleton has as important a role as calcium does. In osteoporosis there is a loss of both components, eventually leading to weakness of the bone structure. A good analogy would be a concrete building, where the combination of both iron rods and cement are necessary for the strength and flexibility of the structure; lack of either could lead to a collapse of the building.

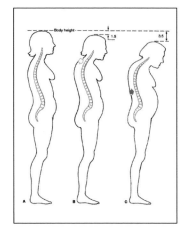

The use of calcium for the prevention of osteoporosis appears to be most important at an early age. Young girls who supplement their calcium intake can increase their bone mass, reducing the chances for bone loss later in life. This concept is very important since some studies suggest that ten to fifteen percent of women younger than thirty may already suffer from osteopenia, an early stage of osteoporosis. The causes for the early bone loss are not clear yet, but it ranges from dietary fads such as lack of dairy products or ultra low fat diets (fat is an essential component for the production of many hormones) to too much exercise (such as jogging several hours a day). The maximum bone mass a woman will ever develop is reached at the end of her growing phase, in her late teens, and it gradually declines from then on; if a woman misses the chance to store calcium in the bones during that period, she will likely start her declining years at a disadvantage.

Vitamin D is another essential component for the health of the bones; lack of it may cause rickets, once a common childhood disease characterized by bone weakness. The metabolism and production of this vitamin in the body is largely dependent on the amount of sunlight that reaches the skin, and people who don't get enough light exposure may need to supplement it with tablets of vitamin D. Use caution and engage the help of your doctor if you suspect a problem since neither too much sun nor excessive vitamin D are good for you.

For reasons that are still not well understood, osteoporosis affects predominantly postmenopausal women, indicating perhaps the strong protection exerted by the estrogen-progesterone duo. Early

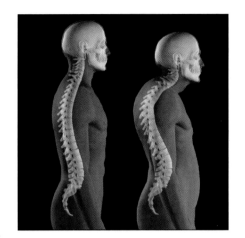

menopause or surgical removal of the ovaries hastens the development of osteoporosis; therefore, women known to have hormonal deficiency must be tested for bone loss at an earlier age than their counterparts. Hormonal replacement has been advocated for years to delay osteoporosis in women who lack it, but recent studies have blamed hormone replacement therapy (HRT) as potentially dangerous in terms of cancer and cardiovascular disease. The choice to use HRT is a personal one, and it needs to be assessed by the woman and her doctor, balancing the risks and the potential lifestyle benefits that many women claim to have from HRT including disappearance of hot flashes, improvement in mood, and enhanced libido, to cite a few. Just to put things in perspective while you make a decision about HRT, remember that hot flashes are temporary, but osteoporosis is permanent.

Healthy men are not immune to developing hormone related osteoporosis since testosterone, the male hormone, is very important in preserving the bone structure. Andropause is the male counterpart of a woman's menopause, and it is associated not only with fatigue, decreased sexual performance, and reduced muscle mass but also with osteoporosis. Men with low testosterone therefore often appear tired and may display thin muscles, decreased body hair, and a slouched posture due to bone loss. The health of both men and women depend on the lifelong cycles of hormones, but both sexes are affected differently from their respective hormonal changes; for example, men get bald sooner than women, but females get osteoporosis at an earlier age.

Although much has been said and written regarding hip fractures in women, about one-fourth of all hip fractures actually occur in men, many times with devastating consequences. Males are more likely to engage in risky behaviors that can lead to fractures and are also less likely to be checked for bone density. Additionally, men tend to consume substantially more alcohol than women, and because of ethanol's toxic effects on the bones, alcoholic men are more prone to develop osteoporosis.

Risk Factors for Osteoporosis

Same as cancer, heart disease, and all other human illnesses, the chances that a person may develop osteoporosis depend on the interaction between one's predisposing factors, such as the DNA we carry and the environment we live in. The list below is the closest to an osteoporosis crystal ball we presently have.

Being Caucasian

White individuals, as well as Asians, have substantially higher chances for age-related bone loss than African-Americans, who seem to have a built-in protection against osteoporosis. This is probably the result of their particular genetic makeup, not the skin color itself. While the body needs sunlight for the manufacture of vitamin D, tanning does not confer any protection against bone loss.

Being Too Thin

Bone mass is particularly sensitive to one's weight: the lighter the person, the more likely the bones are to weaken with age. As a natural response of the skeleton to the effects of gravity, the more weight one (reasonably) exerts on the bones, the stronger they become. Therefore, most obese people are better protected against age related bone loss, while painfully thin people or astronauts who are forced into long periods of weightlessness may develop substantial bone mass reduction. Before you decide to abandon your diet in favor of a heavier frame, notice that obese people are much more likely to suffer from osteoarthritis of the hips and knees, not a great advantage over osteoporosis.

Eating disorders such as bulimia and anorexia carry an even bigger risk to the bones than just being thin, since in addition to the unusually low body weight, these people also suffer from poor nutrition. The loss of electrolytes, calcium, protein, and other nutrients may permanently impair the body's strength, in particular when it occurs during an adolescent's growth period. The damaged skin, hair, and teeth found in girls who suffer from chronic eating disorders are nothing but a reflection of the damage to the internal organs of the body induced by malnutrition, bones and muscles included, which is not as readily apparent to the eye.

Scientist's newly acquired knowledge about the physiology of the body and its response to the force of earth's gravity has direct implications for the design of a fitness plan. For instance, a successful exercise program for posture improvement and osteoporosis prevention must include ways to safely increase the weight load to the spine and long bones, such as by carrying backpacks or weighted vests while walking; this triggers the body's response to strengthen the skeleton. Equally effective, resistive exercises that utilize barbells, elastic bands, and exercise machines can be used to add positive stress to the bones.

Cortisone

The excessive and/or prolonged use of steroids of the kind used to treat inflammation has long been recognized as a cause of bone and muscle loss. One must not confuse these anti-inflammatory steroids with anabolic steroids, which are frequently misused by some athletes to enhance physical performance.

Cortisone can be used orally, as in the treatment of arthritis and poison ivy, or injected in specific areas of the body such as the joints; it does eventually spread to the whole skeleton where it may cause osteoporosis, mainly in the spine. While occasional use of even high doses of cortisone is unlikely to cause medical problems in healthy people, chronic use can and does lead to osteoporosis, hypertension, diabetes, and a number of other ailments.

It is recommended that people who must take regular doses of cortisone undergo studies such as bone density earlier and more frequently than their counterparts. There are several drugs in a pharmacological class called biphosphonates, used in the treatment of osteoporosis, which can also slow down the bone loss due to the use of steroids.

Smoking

Despite the many known health concerns regarding tobacco, a substantial segment of the population still uses it. Nicotine is one of the most addicting substances known, and many individuals who are otherwise intelligent and knowledgeable about the negative health effects of tobacco continue to utilize it.

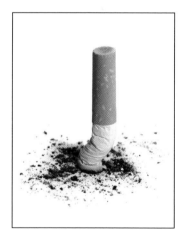

The effects of smoking on the cardiovascular system have been well documented but so has its deleterious action on the musculoskeletal system. The chemicals in tobacco substantially affect collagen, one among the principal components that maintain the integrity of the body. Smoking causes irreversible damage to the connective tissue that makes up the joints, ligaments, and muscles, easily witnessed in the premature wrinkling of the skin of smokers.

Another proof of the damaging effect of smoking on bone integrity is found when testing the ability of bone fractures to heal: smokers are three times more likely to develop a non-union, a weakening of the bone due to incomplete welding of the fractured parts, which may require surgery to correct the subsequent pain and deformity of the limb.

Alcohol

The ingestion of small amounts of alcohol, such as one glass of wine at dinner, appear to have a positive effect on the cardiovascular system, helping prevent heart attacks and reducing the incidence of strokes without a negative effect on bone metabolism. In fact, there is some evidence that drinking small amounts of alcohol may even reduce the incidence of osteoporosis. Drinking large amounts of alcohol, however, is a major cause of osteoporosis not only for men but also for women. Besides having a direct influence on bone function, high alcohol consumption has profound effects on the ability of the liver to metabolize certain chemicals, among them hormones, which are themselves fundamental for bone health.

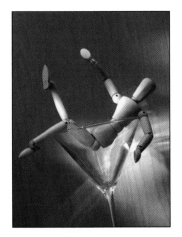

Chronic, excessive alcohol use carries another hidden danger for people already prone to osteoporosis, in the form of nerve damage to the lower extremities. This so called alcoholic peripheral neuropathy causes numbness in the feet and legs with consequent loss of balance, leading to frequent falls, thus greatly enhancing the chances for fractures.

Cola Drinks

Several studies suggest that some carbonated drinks are a risk factor for osteoporosis. The gradual replacement of breakfast milk with diet sodas, which has taken place over the past few years, has been postulated as a possible cause of reduced bone mass in girls. The research, which centers mostly on cola drinks (the ones containing phosphoric acid) continues, and so does the debate. Theoretically, this chemical can alter the proper balance of calcium in the blood, leading to loss of bone strength. Until this issue is settled, it is recommended that the consumption of cola beverages be kept to a minimum.

Family History

Inheritance is one of the strongest predicting factors for osteoporosis: if your mom has it, you too may get it. Open the old photo album and look at the pictures of your grandmother and other female relatives for clues of your own future. Don't assume a fatalistic attitude if your genetic background is not perfect; instead, be pro-active and pay attention to the other treatable risk factors, and insist on obtaining a baseline bone density from your doctor to use as future comparison.

Lack Of Physical Activity

"Use it or lose it" applies to the strength of one's bones as much as it applies to muscles; any bone subjected to the stress of exercises responds by increasing its thickness. Even to the untrained eye, one can detect the effect of exercise on bone strength simply by looking at the dominant arm of a tennis player, thicker and denser than the opposite side.

Inactivity rapidly induces loss of muscle and bone mass, as witnessed by anyone who ever had to wear a cast or by people subjected to long periods in bed due to illness. Immobility can be a catastrophic experience for older folks, who may never fully recover from an otherwise benign condition because of the accelerated brittleness induced by protracted bed rest.

Because of our improved understanding of musculo-skeletal physiology, the medical treatment of injuries and fractures has changed dramatically over the past 25 years. For example, much more emphasis has been placed on early rehabilitative exercises in cases of surgery or trauma. When patients with acute back pain were once told to refrain from walking and ambulating for several weeks to give the spine time to rest, we now push for early rehabilitation to avoid worsening of the symptoms due to the inevitable bone and muscle atrophy that results from inactivity.

Summary

Our crystal ball suggests that the most likely person to develop osteoporosis is a white, thin, postmenopausal, non-exercising, smoking, cola-sipping, alcohol-drinking woman, with a positive family history. On the plus side, the only risk factor she can't do anything about is her genetic makeup.

Standing Tall –
Your Posture Fitness Program

Getting Started

Humans have an amazing capacity to find excuses for their actions and to rationalize even the most outrageous behavior (and that doesn't apply just to teenagers). When asked if they exercise regularly, many people reply: "I walk plenty at work," or "I don't have a membership to a gym," or "I just hate exercising." It is not uncommon for a person to overestimate the amount of physical activity accomplished during their everyday chores, thus justifying the lack of a separate fitness routine. Some of us incorrectly believe that cookie crumbs have no calories; others trust that walking down the hall "a hundred times a day" really does qualify as a workout.

Don't feel guilty if you don't enjoy exercising; I know very few people who actually do. Even avid exercisers like myself will tell you that they dread getting started on their daily fitness program, but this initial reluctance gradually decreases after the first few minutes of exercise. Afterwards, at the end of an exercise routine, most people will feel energized, accomplished, alert, and happier.

This book is divided into sections according to the muscle groups, exercise modalities, and equipment utilized. The last chapter carries a compilation of several different routines, mixing and matching various exercises to suit specific fitness goals for people of different physical capacities, ages, and general status. Utilize it as basic guide, and use your own creativity to design a program that works for you.

While there is no such thing as a fitness routine that will make a person taller, the proper contraction and relaxation of specific muscle groups in a regimented fitness program permits the spine to stretch and allows us to reach our maximum height.

Exercise is an Investment

In a world of uncertainty, there are few things that have as predictable a pay-off, as reliable an outcome, as a fitness program. The vast majority of people who enroll in an exercise routine will eventually obtain appreciable physical and mental benefits from it. Despite the obvious gains in health and improved quality of life, many of us choose to take better care of our "stuff" than our own bodies. From polishing the silverware to changing the oil in the car, we devote a substantial amount of time to less important items than our own health, assuming that somehow our bodies

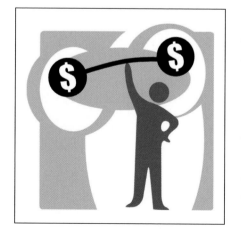

will take care of themselves. That's not so, and I remind the reader about the needless hours people must wait at doctor's offices and the many diseases which could be improved or prevented by maintaining an exercise program. The benefits from exercising include: blood pressure reduction, weight loss, depression relief, diabetes prevention, and osteoporosis avoidance, just to cite a few. The resources you spend exercising will later be recouped, with interest, in potential time and money that would otherwise be wasted with lost work, doctors appointments, and painful procedures.

The Best Time of the Day to Exercise

There's no absolute best time to exercise; it depends on the needs of the individual doing it. You may choose to exercise based on your specific time constraints from work, home, or school, or you may want to select the time based on your biorhythm, that is, the time of the day when you either have the most energy, or when you need it the most. For example, morning people, those whose combination of hormones, temperature, and brain chemicals peak early in the day, may select going to the gym immediately after waking up, enjoying the extra vigor to push themselves in the direction of the gym. Or instead, they may save the exercises for later, as an antidote 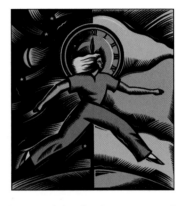 to the fatigue that creeps in by the middle of the afternoon and spoils the rest of the day for so many of us. Anyway, avoid working out too late in the evening since exercising before going to bed may impair one's sleep.

If your health permits it, try to perform the whole exercise routine in a single sitting instead of splitting it into two or more sessions spread out during the day. If you must split your routine, do so by clustering them according to type: stretching, aerobic, and resistive. It is important to maintain an elevated heart rate for a substantial part of an aerobic program in order to obtain the maximum cardiac benefit; during the anaerobic part of that program the benefits are greatest when the muscles develop fatigue and have to resort to energy produced by alternative metabolic pathways.

Going go the Gym versus Home Exercises

It takes a lot of discipline to carry a regular exercise program at home. Although at first it seems easier than going to a gym, it can quickly become lonely and boring. Humans are, after all, social animals that benefit from group interaction at many different levels, including engaging in positive behavior from peer pressure. When surrounded by other people who are themselves exercising, we are more likely to complete our own fitness routine, aware that someone next to us will perhaps be paying attention if we give up after the first few repetitions. The prompt availability of a wide range of exercise machines at the gym, already in place and just begging to be utilized, tends to increase the likelihood that one's daily workout will be completed.

Whether exercising at home or going to the gym, set aside the time for the full routine, don't do it just when you have an "opening." Try not to stop for a quick break on your way to the gym, or you may end up skipping it altogether. Save the pre-exercise latte or the candy bar for later, as a reward for a job well done.

Headphones and some up-tempo music do add some lively energy to an otherwise lackluster fitness routine and may help you squeeze out a few extra repetitions. Reading or watching TV during your workout can overcome boredom during an aerobic routine. Books on tape may work well for someone who feels that the time "wasted" on staying fit should be better spent. Reading a book or magazine while using a stationary bike is considered safe, but doing it while exercising on a treadmill may cause dizziness or loss of balance and should be done cautiously, if at all.

Despite the fact that some physical fitness instructors advise their trainees that total concentration on the exercises is necessary to obtain maximum benefits, I have not seen convincing proof of that. I suspect that daydreaming during one's workout routine generates as much physical benefit as grunting through the exercises; as for myself, I often let my mind wander to my "happy place" while my body is engaged in "auto pilot."

> Tip: if you perspire a lot, choose an exercise location in the gym directly underneath one of the air conditioning vents.

Do I Need an Exercise Buddy?

A lot depends on how motivated you are. Exercising with another person may provide the enthusiasm needed to start and maintain a fitness program; both of you may gain from the benign harassing and teasing that friends normally do to each other, and it will increase compliance with the exercises. Companionship and competitiveness are a plus, and a buddy allows for exercises that require two people for their execution. Couples may find that the time spent working out together enhances their ability to communicate.

Instead of exercising with a buddy, some people choose to do it in front of the mirror, challenging their alter ego, demanding from himself or herself one more squat or one more sit up. There is nothing wrong if you catch yourself talking to your reflection, cajoling and encouraging that person facing you in the mirror to push the exercises further. If you possess even a trace of vanity, a mirror can be your best friend and ally to encourage you to keep a proper posture.

Hydration

As kids we learn about the consistency of blood from the inevitable cuts and bruises we suffer while growing up. Not as thin as water, not as thick as oil, blood's viscosity is a reflection of its composition: serum (the liquid part) diluting the red cells, white cells, and platelets (the solid part). Blood needs to be thin enough to go through the microscopic capillary vessels of the lungs, kidneys, and the rest of the body. Any substantial loss of fluids during exercises makes the blood thicker and its flow more difficult, with consequent repercussions to the body unless continuous replenishment of the lost liquid normalizes the viscosity. The heart initially compensates for the decreased fluid and the thicker blood by working harder and pumping faster; eventually, dehydration causes a collapse of the circulatory system, dropping the blood pressure enough to cause fainting, or worse.

Not only do one's heart, lungs, and muscles become less efficient when there is significant fluid loss, but the kidneys can't filter properly either, a grim prospect considering that strenuous exercises can release substantial quantities of myoglobin, a common muscle protein, into the bloodstream. Myoglobin needs plenty of fluid to allow its filtration and elimination by the kidneys at the risk of clogging the microscopic filters responsible for the production of urine. Marathon runners and professional athletes are familiar with the occasional passing of red tinted urine, colored by myoglobin, following an exhausting competition.

As a rule of thumb, try to drink a few ounces of liquid before you start your workout; don't wait until you become thirsty to start replenishing fluids since it is common for a "pumped-up" exerciser to disregard the body's initial dehydration warnings. This becomes even more vital if you're doing a strenuous workout in a hot environment, when the body may lose water faster than it can absorb. Remember that if you do become dehydrated, you can develop nausea and vomiting, making it difficult or impossible to regain the lost volume of fluid by ingestion alone.

Plain water is the liquid of choice to replenish the body fluids in all but the most strenuous activities. Gatorade or similar beverages may have an advantage in limited circumstances, like during some long, arduous, sun drenched workouts, because it replenishes both lost electrolytes and calories.

Despite a flood of ads that promote specially formulated light beer for "physically active people," alcohol is an obviously poor choice as an exercise drink and should be avoided for at least a couple of hours before or after exercising due to its dehydrating properties and negative effect on coordination. Dieters should note that alcohol contains seven calories per gram, almost fifty percent more than pure sugar!

The jury is still divided as to whether coffee has any negative effect on exercising. Limiting caffeine consumption to no more than 100-200 mg. is sensible and probably OK for most people despite some increase in heart rate.

> Tip: older people may have an impaired sense of thirst and can easily become dehydrated because they "forget" to replenish the liquids they lose. The ingestion of six to eight glasses of fluid distributed throughout the day is a reasonable preventive measure; still, the most reliable way to detect dehydration in an otherwise healthy person is when there is reduced urine production, such as when Grandma has not used the bathroom "all day long."

What to Wear

Shoes

Proper shoes are a must, not just for exercising, but also for everyday use to prevent possible damage to our precious feet and ankles. Tennis shoes, although not suitable for every occasion, are still the best

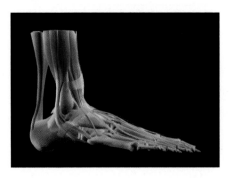 bet provided that they are: a) wide enough at the base to stabilize the ankle and keep you from developing sprains, and b) cushioned at the heel to reduce the chances for spurs or plantar fasciitis, both very painful conditions. Don't forget that, as you age, the feet widen due to laxity of the ligaments that normally would hold the bones tightly together; you also lose some of the "springiness" of the gait due to the loss of the normal curvature of the foot arch. Don't just buy the same size shoes you've always worn (one's feet never stop growing), try them for fit and comfort allowing for the inevitable changes that have occurred with age, such as bunions and calluses. Special orders can be placed for hard to find sizes, while custom-made inserts should be utilized in limited cases and by prescription. You don't need to buy an expensive,

trendy tennis shoe, but you should avoid purchasing the flimsiest ones since the poor construction and substandard materials usually employed in these models are unlikely to provide the support you need.

Clothes

Workout clothes must be selected by where and when you plan to exercise. At home, it may even be optional if you don't mind some bouncing, scratches, and the inevitable rug burn. Instead of wearing an old cotton T-shirt and jogging pants, you may prefer to create the right exercise environment by choosing clothes similar to what you would wear at the gym.

Both men and women may prefer to wear workout clothes made from one of the modern breathable fibers that carries sweat away from the skin and allows for rapid evaporation when perspiring. If you have sensitive skin, choose your outfit fabric wisely since any material that feels itchy when dry can become much itchier when damp. The addition of loose shorts worn as outerwear over skin-hugging gym clothes may allow you more freedom and modesty to perform your exercise routine, and it usually conforms better to the dressing code in most health clubs.

Underwear

Women, well endowed or not, must wear a sports bra for support and comfort. Don't skimp on this item since a good bra aids in proper posture and reduces the unsightly and uncomfortable bouncing. Larger breasts require more support and you should avoid buying them too small or it may make breathing more difficult during exercises. Once you find a good bra, buy two of them to make sure you'll always have a clean, dry one to wear; get new ones every few months since they lose their effectiveness after repeated use due to stretching. Be attentive to the underwear you use since it tends to show more through damp clothes.

Men should wear supportive underwear while exercising because it cuts down on chafing, and it reduces the chances of trauma or torsion of the testicles, a very painful condition at best.

The Exercise Trio

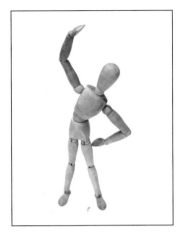

Any decent fitness program consists of a combination of stretching, aerobic, and anaerobic exercises. Remove one leg from this tripod and the whole program falls. Stretching elongates the muscles, ligaments, and tendons in a way that permits the other two elements of the program to provide maximum benefit. The term aerobic refers to the utilization of oxygen by the muscle to produce the energy necessary for its contraction during mild to moderate physical activity. On the other hand, strenuous, vigorous exercises, such as weight training, can't be accomplished using oxygen alone, and the muscles employ other chemical means to produce the required amount of energy: an anaerobic system. Unfortunately this anaerobic pathway runs out of steam quickly and can't be sustained for extended periods of time. That's why slow paced exercises like walking can be done continuously but weight lifting can't since it requires quick bursts of extra energy.

Walking and Weight Bearing

As one of the most common forms of aerobic training, walking can be a fun proposition when the weather is nice, and it is certainly excellent for the cardio respiratory system and for the health of the joints. When properly done, it is a first-rate form of posture training, but when utilized alone, walking is a poor exercise option for osteoporosis prevention. Unless additional tension is applied to the skeleton, the bones are unlikely to benefit much from a plain walking program, and they may fail to incorporate a substantial amount of calcium to their structure.

A good trick to enhance your workout consists in carrying a few extra pounds while walking, either by holding hand weights, or, better yet, by carrying a backpack. One can add weight to the backpack in the form of plastic water bottles, which can be emptied at any time if they become too heavy. As an alternative, water-carrying backpacks, such as the ones utilized by bikers and hikers, may provide not only the weight to power your stroll, but will also supply hydrating fluids during long walks. This weight carrying method loads the spine and the long bones of the body, like the femur, with the added tension and stress necessary for bone strengthening.

In order to avoid the low back pain that can arise from carrying too much weight over one's shoulders, some people may be better served by utilizing a weighted belt around the waist, therefore sparing excessive stress over the lower back, and though it loads the bones in the lower extremities, it won't help prevent osteoporosis of the spine.

Aquatic Exercises

Water therapy is an excellent exercise modality, but it should be regarded as only one part of a more comprehensive posture program because it does not challenge the skeletal system with enough weight or resistance. Nevertheless, everyone except the very frail can do an aerobic water workout since it carries little chance of injuries. For those who prefer to swim, it is indeed among the best aerobic exercises one can do, and it helps develop the trunk muscles responsible for proper posture. People with neck problems may prefer to wear a mask and snorkel while swimming, in order to avoid rotating or overextending the cervical spine when surfacing to breathe.

Will I Get Too Muscular?

What a difference a century makes: well to do people in the early 1900's abhorred suntans and strong muscles because these were the hallmarks of farmers and manual laborers, symbols of a lower class status. Now we spend billions on fitness while most gyms make tanning beds and sprays available to complement the perfect, sexy body.

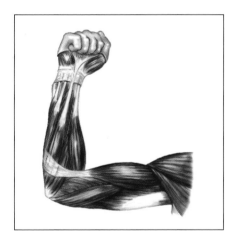

Although most men tend to welcome any and all boost to their muscle mass, many women feel that an increase in the size of their muscles will make them look less feminine. While this may be correct in the case of young females who strive for the delicate, waif, fragile look, the opposite holds true for most women, especially as they mature. A stronger physique will not only keep aging structures from sagging, but as a universal marker for health, well-delineated muscles will visually counterbalance many of the other signs of aging, such as wrinkles or skin spots. Great biceps and deltoids, for example, will make your arms look younger than their chronological years.

As age progresses, it becomes more difficult to maintain strong, solid muscles. Over the years, we steadily lose muscle mass due to, according to some scientists, certain proteins produced by our own body, which appear to be toxic to the muscles. Strange as it sounds, it is important to realize that this is not just a passive loss of muscle from idleness but an active chemical process that little by little subtracts from the muscles. On average, it causes a healthy person to lose half a pound of muscle per year after age thirty-five. Sufficient exercises are therefore needed to develop a net muscle gain, a difficult task at best, made even more difficult while fighting arthritis and other age related problems.

The challenge we face in that muscle tug-of-war reminds me of Penelope's Web, the story of the Greek queen Penelope, who waited ten years for the return of her husband Ulysses. She postponed choosing a suitor to replace the missing king until she had finished sewing an intricate web; she secretly undid at night what she sewed during the day, awaiting for Ulysses' return. We lose muscles so fast as we age that one could say, exaggerating just a little, that we lose at night the muscles we build during the day.

How To Avoid Getting Injured

Assuming that no major illness exists that would require a doctor's release before exercising, start low and go slow. Be aware that your prior physical status will dictate what kind of program you should follow. Throughout the book you'll find recommendations regarding modified exercises that could apply to you. We recommend a program with three days of exercise a week as the bare minimum. Less than that and you become more prone to injuries.

It is not uncommon to experience pain and soreness during the initial days of a fitness program. At a microscopic level, the increase in strength and stamina obtained from a workout occurs when the muscle cells repair and rebuild themselves after being strained and damaged by exercises. The local release of chemicals by the muscle aids in its repair, but it takes several hours after completing a particular exercise for the production and release of these agents. These chemicals not only help in the healing process but also cause temporary pain and inflammation; therefore, one does not usually develop aching muscles and joints until a day later. Remember this before deciding on a sudden, sizeable increase in your routine of exercises just because you're having a good day.

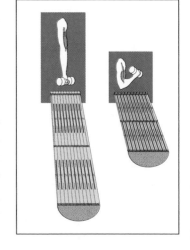

The "no pain, no gain" maxim should be followed with caution since a certain burning feeling and pain in the muscles is to be expected if they are to become stronger, while pain in the joints and tendons could indicate a more serious problem due to damage and chronic inflammation. It seems that the difference between good pain and bad pain lies principally in the ability of the tissues to heal: tendons and joints heal very slowly and therefore they are more apt to suffer from new injuries before the old ones are cured.

After reading the previous chapters, one can better understand why the body's capacity for healing decreases with age, but science can only partially explain why children have such an enormous ability for quick healing while older people do not. Injuries to both young and old exercisers can be avoided simply by using good sense, pacing, and sticking to a routine until one feels strong enough to add to it. Becoming impatient with what seems to be too slow a progress is a sure path to injury.

Any injury should be followed by a few days resting the affected area either by discontinuing the workout routine completely or by modifying it enough to allow healing to occur. A common mistake injured exercisers make is to try to catch-up with lost time by quickly resuming a full program, erroneously assuming that once the pain improves, the injury itself should be cured. This often leads to a pattern of recurring injuries, interrupted by a few days of partial rest and resulting in chronic painful conditions, such as tendonitis and arthritis.

A great way to stay fit during recovery is to exercise in a swimming pool, not only for the buoyancy that unloads the weight from the joints but also for the resistance imposed by the water which does not allow for sudden movements of a painful limb. If an injured lower extremity is swollen, great benefit may result from walking inside the pool because the weight and pressure of the water increase with depth, being maximal at the feet and minimal at the surface, resulting in a natural, painless, graduated compression of the legs that eventually pushes the fluid from a swollen leg back to the circulatory system.

Agonist and Antagonist Muscles

For every movable joint in the body, there are two opposing muscle groups: the agonist, which moves the segment of the body in one direction and the antagonist, which moves it in the opposite direction. For example, the biceps and the triceps muscles have opposing effects, one flexing and the other extending the arm. A good fitness program requires that the workout include exercises for both agonists and antagonists to achieve proper balance. This is not intuitive, and many adults who do exercise on a regular basis often do it improperly, excessively favoring a specific muscle group during their workout in order to acquire a desirable body feature.

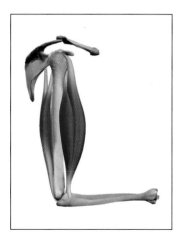

That's the case of the *Six Pack Syndrome*, a term that I use to describe the overuse of abdominal exercises through sit-ups, crunches, and specialized workout equipment in order to obtain a glamorous and sexy abdominal rectus muscle, the coveted "six-pack." Working the abdominal muscles without developing the corresponding posterior trunk muscles is a common and grave workout error, which may lead to back pain, excessive stooping, and an exaggerated forward curvature of the spine due to the ensuing muscle tone imbalance.

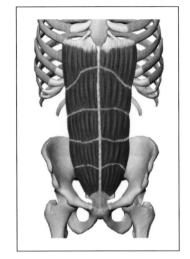

By the way, it is next to impossible to produce a great "six-pack" through abdominal exercises alone; one must also trim down any excess body fat, including the kind that accumulates around the waist and obstructs the muscle in question from view. You don't believe me? Just look at any adolescent skinny boy with less than twelve percent body fat to verify the presence of an effortless "six-pack."

Advice for Injury Prevention

Lower Back

Even healthy people may suffer from back pain. If one realizes that the lumbar spine resting just above the pelvis holds all of the weight of the head, arms, and trunk and that, despite that heavy load, we still require that it be able to bend and twist, it is amazing that there is anybody at all who does not suffer from back pain.

Each of the vertebrae that make up the spine behaves like a tripod with a thick front leg resting on the disk that separates and cushions the bones in the spine and two smaller hind legs that join similar protrusions from bones above and below it. All of that is held in place by a complex system of ligaments and some of the strongest muscles in the body.

Close attention needs to be paid to the correct spinal alignment when exercising since any deviation from the right position will be magnified by the effects of gravity or the use of weights. While a torn muscle usually heals nicely, a disk tear never heals and often remains a source of intermittently severe pain for years. Since it is so ubiquitous, many people choose not to seek medical help for their lower back problems, but any pain that radiates to the lower extremity (or the upper extremity when it is the neck that is involved) indicates a possible nerve compromise and needs attention from a health care professional.

Shoulders

A bit of trivia for those not familiar with the anatomy of the shoulder: it barely qualifies as a joint. If you put a tennis ball on the open palm of your hand you get a good approximation of what the joint looks like, a structure held in place due only to the strong, specialized ligaments and tendons that surround it. The same construction that gives the shoulder the ability to move in such a wide range of directions is also

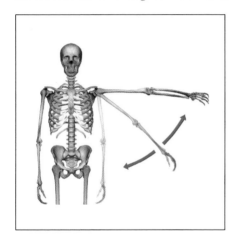

its downfall, making it rather unstable and prone to injuries, dislocations, and inflammation. Due to biomechanical constraints, the unit that comprises the shoulder joint, including the ligaments that hold it in place and the muscles that allow it to move, works best and safest when one refrains from reaching the extreme ranges while performing exercises. For example, lifting one's arms sideways beyond ninety degrees, while holding weights, doesn't add much to the workout but it greatly increases the chances for damage; the same occurs when allowing the arms and elbows to reach too far back while using a butterfly machine.

As a rule, the farther in any direction the elbows are from the trunk, the bigger the chances that injuries will occur to the shoulder; furthermore, these chances increase exponentially as heavier weights are used while exercising. Because of the leverage exerted from even small weights held away from the body, an action apparently as simple as reaching back to pick a briefcase from the backseat of a car could damage some of the ligaments and tendons that sustain the shoulder, possibly causing a tear to the structure we call rotator cuff.

Knees

The knees are wonderful, sturdy joints that allow us to run, climb, and kick, but the knees also have a dark side for they contain a self-destructive mode: it's called twisting. The mechanism is comparable to what occurs to two pieces of metal joined by a single droplet of superglue; despite a formidable resistance to pulling forces, they can easily be separated by twisting them apart. The upper and the lower halves of the knees are held in place not by glue, but by strands of connective tissue: ligaments that run in a criss-cross fashion. Although the knees are strong enough to tolerate years of severe daily beatings from a jogger, it takes only an instant for a foot stuck in a hole and a twisting motion of the body for the ligaments to snap.

Good shoes and a flat surface go a long way in preventing injuries. Keep both feet on the ground when the exercise allows for it. Avoid the excessive stress that may result from exercising with the knees bent beyond ninety degrees, as it adds very little to the exercise and greatly increases the possibility of damage. Exercise cautiously, if at all, when the knee hurts, or if it is red or swollen.

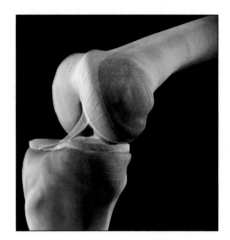

As Long as You're At It...

Most people get involved in a fitness program because they want to improve the quality of their lives. Since a suitable state of mind geared for health improvement already exists, one might also consider other lifestyle changes, including weight loss when appropriate, better stress management, or quitting cigarettes.

Smoking cessation is particularly difficult, and there are as many different methods to quit smoking as there are smokers, from acupuncture to antidepressants. Whatever the option one chooses to quit the use of tobacco, one thing is certain: no method works unless the person is ready to quit. A good starting point is to prohibit oneself from smoking in any enclosed location, such as at home or in the car. Making it less convenient to light up reduces the number of units smoked, and the decline in the re-breathing of indoor smoke particles is an added bonus. Restraining any and all smoking from common areas such as one's home may also make it easier if only one of the spouses from a couple that smokes wishes to quit.

Since smoking is such an entrenched addiction, the brain will find inexhaustible excuses for a person to continue to "enjoy" nicotine, such as using it to "soothe" the nerves because one has had a hard day at work. If you need a plan to quit, you can try a rigid program that limits the number of cigarettes allowed on a twenty-four hour period, reducing it by a pre-determined number. For example, try decreasing the total number of cigarettes smoked, reducing the daily maximum each week by one, thus avoiding many of the symptoms of withdrawal. If you can't make it on your own, ask your doctor about oral medications or patches to help you quit. Remember that smoking is a major risk factor for osteoporosis.

Weight loss is one of the main incentives for obese people to exercise, and there are varied explanations for the weight loss observed. Not only does an exercise routine burn calories at a higher rate, but it will also decrease hunger for one to two hours afterwards; therefore, finishing one's fitness program just before dinnertime is a natural appetite suppressant and an added bonus to any weight loss program. Exercises also reduce anxiety and the need to consume "comfort foods," and it may help stabilize blood sugar levels.

Don't get hung up on what the bathroom scale shows when you start a fitness program. It is not uncommon for a person to lose one or two pounds of excess fat per week while exercising, but some fluid retention or loss may occur at first, depending on the individual, and it may translate into inaccurate weight readings. Many times the scale does not accurately reflect the true health benefits gained from exercising because as fat is burned and muscles are strengthened, the body becomes denser, more compact, thus a person is more likely to notice a reduction in dress or pant sizes, rather than a huge amount of weight loss.

Life stressors are unavoidable, but the way we choose to deal with anxiety can be modified. Stress management is a term widely used but poorly defined; it essentially refers to one's ability to control and reduce the body's harmful reaction to life's negative events. For instance, stress can cause a massive release of potent chemicals, such as adrenaline and cortisol into the bloodstream with a significant impact on the heart, blood vessels, and the brain itself. Exercises, on the other hand, can be such powerful stress reducers that psychiatrists often recommend a fitness program as part of the therapy for people with mild depression before embarking on a regimen of drugs.

Interestingly, women seem to be more susceptible than men to the positive effects that exercises have on mood to the point that sudden discontinuation of daily exercises can cause symptoms similar to drug withdrawal, with generalized aches, fatigue, and depression. When appropriate, we recommend that both women and men continue to exercise the unaffected parts of the body after an injury to avoid the withdrawal feeling from sudden exercise discontinuation. Exercising the upper part of the body in case of a leg fracture, or taking up swimming after a low back injury that prevents other aerobic routines, are examples of adequate fitness substitutions.

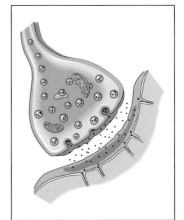

Pain and the profound physiologic effects exerted on it by exercises have been well documented, both in humans as well as animals. For example, athletes who get injured during a game may remain unaware of the severity of their condition until the competition is over. Endorphins are the small morphine-like molecules that are frequently cited as the brain chemicals responsible for this pain blockade, but the scientific data is still wanting. Other substances may also be involved, including cortisol, the natural steroid hormone, which is released during fight-or-flight situations. Independent of which brain chemicals are responsible for exercise-induced analgesia, a fitness program remains one of the main therapies for chronic painful conditions, such as fibromyalgia and osteoarthritis.

Customizing Your Workout

It would literally take a person several hours to execute all of the exercises contained in this book. Then again, it wouldn't make any more sense to follow this book, page by page, than it would be to cook all of the recipes in a kitchen book. I suggest that first you browse through the exercises, making a mental note as to the ones that would be most appropriate for you, before embarking on your program. You'll notice that many of the exercises are variations of a common theme, each with an additional degree of difficulty in their execution.

One modification that can easily be done and is often used by hard-core exercisers is the so-called Around The World routine. You may apply it, for instance, to the lunges or to the Swiss ball routines contained in the book. Instead of following each exercise to the letter, you may combine them as exemplified in the exercises on pages 114 and 115, moving through each successive exercise, without going back to the starting position.

"First do no harm," and "Start low and go slow," used to be my mottos in medical school, and I trust they apply here too. A safe way to begin your program is to choose a workout level you think you can perform, but start at one level lower. This means also limiting the weight and number of repetitions, besides choosing the appropriate exercises. At the end of the book, you'll find a few selected workouts we have put together based on the amount of time or physical limitations one may have.

Use this book as a well-intentioned guide, but don't be constrained just by the examples presented here. Try to design your own workout. Mix and match the exercises and create your own personal posture fitness program by following some simple rules:

- Remember to start with a good warm-up.
- Exercises shouldn't hurt.
- Keep a balanced program that uses different muscle groups and avoid favoring the abs over the other core muscles.
- Adjust the number of repetitions of the chosen exercises according to how many similar exercises you have selected.
- Choose the stretches that best complement your workout.
- Be realistic. Rome was not built in a day either.

Warm Up

Before you begin your daily fitness program, you have to warm up. There is no secret formula and no need for specialized equipment; the main goal of a warm-up is to increase the blood flow to the muscles before you demand from them. Cold muscles are prone to injuries and tears, and it renders the exercises more difficult and less productive.

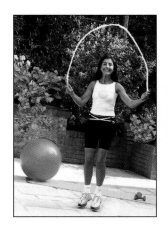

If the weather in your area permits it, choose a warm-up exercise that you can perform outdoors. You don't have to look any further than your own backyard or one of the local parks to enjoy the colors of spring, a crisp autumn morning, or the smell of freshly cut grass.

Walking, swimming, and biking are all very good alternatives, but jumping rope and jumping jacks are unbeatable as the best options when it comes to a warm up that works on your posture. What's so special about both exercises? Not only are they great for warming up before a fitness routine because they recruit and activate all the important muscle groups in the body, but these two wonderful exercises repeatedly load the spine and the long bones of the lower extremities with additional weight during each jump. Thus, they strengthen the bones and reduce the chances for osteoporosis. Jogging is another good weight-loading warm up, but I don't recommend it for most people since the strain on the knees and ankles

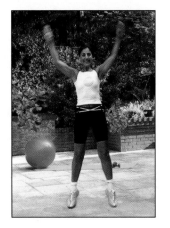

is much greater than jumping in place, and it can more easily lead to injuries or early arthritis.

If you're not obese and you prefer to walk as a warm up, remember that you may benefit from wearing a backpack weighted with a few plastic bottles filled with water to increase your weight. During the summer months you may enjoy having some cold water to drink or just to cool your back. Dump the water if it gets too heavy. Remember to be a little more careful not to fall when carrying a heavy backpack, because the additional weight raises your center of gravity and decreases your stability when walking.

Let's Get Started!

The next ten chapters contain a series of exercises divided according to the equipment and muscle groups utilized for the workouts. Keep in mind that we have included many different variations of each exercise; carefully choose the ones that best match your fitness condition, using the difficulty level guide which accompanies each exercise.

· Safety should be your first priority.

· Fun should be your second priority.

· Start low and go slow.

· Avoid injuries by listening to your body.

· Remember to warm up and stretch.

· When in doubt, ask your doctor before beginning this or any exercise program.

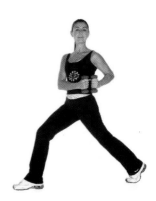

L unges are among the best exercises to enhance one's posture, simple but deceptively difficult to execute properly (you can think of them as controlled falling). Like so many exercises in this book, lunges require patience and repetition to achieve the perfection that maximizes core muscle tone and improves spinal stability.

Lunges increase the muscle tone of the gluteus, quadriceps, and hip flexor muscles while stretching the quadriceps of the rear leg. The addition of hand weights to the routine not only increases the effort of the lower extremities and therefore the gain, but it engages the muscles of the upper extremities and trunk as well. Lowering the height of the hand weights also lowers the body's center of gravity, adding stability and ease to the lunges (think high-wire artist); the opposite, lifting the weights higher, increases the degree of difficulty of the exercises. Begin with the easier exercise variations first until you feel ready to try the more difficult ones.

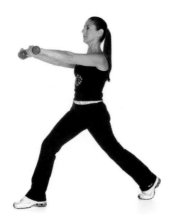

The Forward Arm Raise variation, pictured on the opposite page (and pose 4 on page 46), is the best lunge because the position of the weights shifts the center of gravity of the trunk high up and to the front, thus activating the posterior muscles of the upper, middle, and lower spine, so important for posture maintenance. This particular lunge holds an extra level of difficulty, which is more than rewarded by improving your stance and balance.

Remember: Each exercise is labeled with its difficulty level. Be sure to start with Beginner exercises and build your way to Advanced!

| ●○○ | ●●○ | ●●● |
| Beginner | Medium | Advanced |

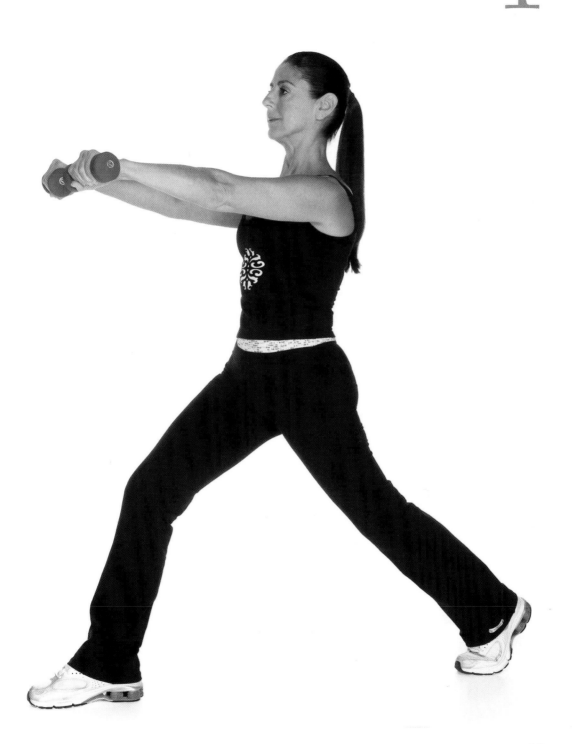

Stretches

No fitness program is complete without proper muscle stretching. Do them preferably after each group of exercises, but you can repeat the stretches any time or in any order you feel your body requires; just listen to your muscles and joints. If it hurts, stop because you've gone too far.

Stretching elongates the muscles, reduces the chances for injuries, and maximizes the gain from your workout.

1 - Quadriceps Stretch

Grab one foot behind you and pull it back until you feel the quadriceps muscle stretching. Gradually elevate the opposite arm while adjusting your balance. Hold for 10-20 seconds and change to the other side.

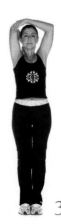
1

2 - Shoulder Stretch

Keep the arm straight and bring it across your body parallel to the ground. Help the movement by pulling in with the other hand and pressing just above the elbow joint. Hold for 10-20 seconds and change to the other side.

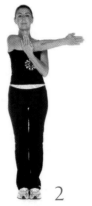
2

3 - Triceps Stretch

Raise your arm and try to touch the spine between your shoulder blades. Use the other hand to pull the elbow in until you feel the triceps muscle stretch. Hold for 10-20 seconds and change to the other side.

3

Hints and Tips:

· *For maximum results, bend the back knee further during your lunges, and never allow the front knee to travel too far forward, past the ankle*

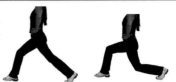

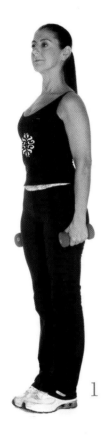

Unless noted otherwise, pose 1 is the starting position for all of the lunge exercises described here. You may choose to do all of them or you may select a few exercises, customizing the workout by adjusting the number of repetitions accordingly.

Each of the lunge variations can be done as described below or they can be performed as an "Around The World" routine, moving from curl to forward raise, lateral raise, and so forth, performing all the different arm movements in succession, keeping the feet firmly planted on the ground. Remember to bend the back knee towards the floor to maximize the exercise.

1 - Initial Position

Start by standing erect with your feet together, looking forward. Firmly hold small to medium size weights in your hands. Remember to roll the shoulders back and down.

●○○

2 - Basic Lunge w/ Weights

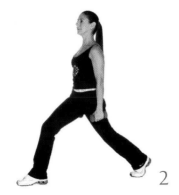

Hold the weights low to your side, take a big step forward, and plant the front foot firmly on the ground, while keeping the back foot stationary. Lower your trunk by partially flexing the knees until you feel the tension in the muscles. Distribute the weight to the heel of the front foot and the toes of the hind foot. Step back to the starting position. Repeat the exercise alternating the right and left legs, 10-20 times each.

 ●○○

3 - Curl

When lunging, flex your biceps and bring the weights up to chest height. Step back to the starting position. Do 10-20 repetitions with each leg.

●○○

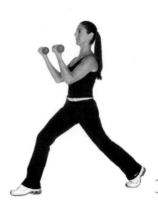

3

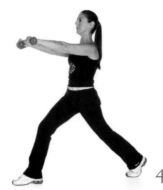

4

4 - Forward Arm Raise

When lunging, lift your arms forward, keeping them straight and parallel to the ground. Step back to the starting position. Do 10-20 repetitions with each leg.

●○○

5 - Lateral Arm Raise

When lunging, lift your arms sideways while flexing your elbows 90 degrees. Step back to the starting position. Do 10-20 repetitions with each leg.

●○○

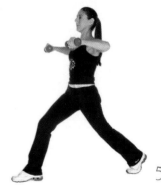

5

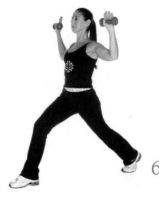

6

6 - Upward Shoulder Rotation

Same as pose 5, but this time, when lunging, flex your elbows 90 degrees and rotate your arms up until the hands reach the height of your ears. Step back to the starting position. Do 10-20 repetitions with each leg.

●○○

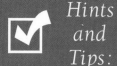

Hints and Tips:

· *Inhale during the start position and exhale during the lunges.*
· *Lower the weights twice as slowly as it took to raise them.*
· *Control is the operative word. Perform the exercise slowly and uniformly, without sudden jerks.*

7 - Overhead Press

Same as pose 5, but this time, when lunging, elevate the weights above your head. Step back to the starting position. Do 10-20 repetitions with each leg.

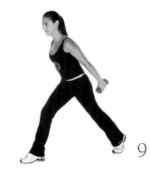

8 - Lunge and Rotate

Start standing up straight. Hold the weights in front of you at waist height by keeping the elbows flexed and to your side. When lunging, rotate your trunk sideways, flex your elbows ninety degrees, and keep the weights close to the abdomen. Step back to the starting position. Do 10-20 repetitions with each leg.

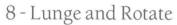

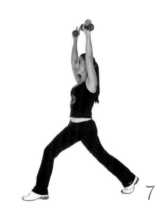

9 - Triceps Extension

Start standing up straight. Hold the weights in front of you at waist height by keeping the elbows flexed and to your side. When lunging, bring the weights behind you by extending the elbows and rotating the shoulders back. Leaning your trunk forward will help you lift the weights higher. Do 10-20 repetitions with each leg.

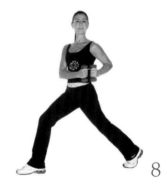

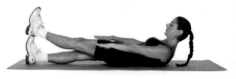

Floor abdominals are one of the basic building blocks of core strength, and yet, no fancy equipment or weights are needed. Instead, the pull of gravity on the arms and legs supply the necessary resistance for a strong work out. Because the muscles in the posterior trunk oppose and balance the abdominal muscles, and together they provide the stability of the spine, it is fundamental that both groups of muscles be exercised to achieve balance. Your posture will suffer if you perform the abdominal work out without exercising the corresponding muscles of the trunk.

Start with the easier exercise variations first until you feel ready to try the more difficult ones.

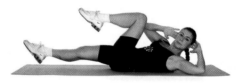

We chose the exercise highlighted on the opposite page, the One-Hundred With Elevated Legs, (and pose 5 on page 52) as the best among the floor abdominal variants and one of the most arduous. The leveraged weight of the legs is supported by the continuous contraction of the anterior abdominal muscles. The repetitive hand motion that gives the exercise its name not only adds power to the exercise but it is also a welcome distraction that eases the discomfort of maintaining the legs elevated for so long.

Remember: Each exercise is labeled with its difficulty level. Be sure to start with Beginner exercises and build your way to Advanced!

⬤◯◯ ⬤⬤◯ ⬤⬤⬤
Beginner   Medium   Advanced

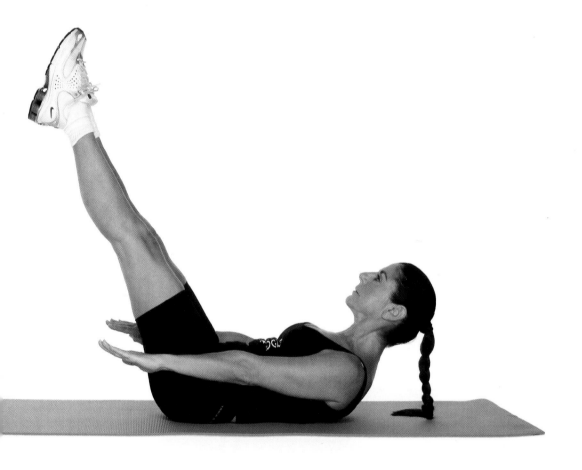

Floor Stretches

1 - Knee to Chest

Sit up, straighten one leg and bend the other one. Hold the knee and bring it towards you for 10-20 seconds. Release and switch.

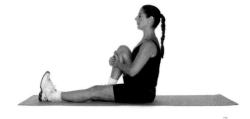

1

2 - Knee Hug

Lying on the floor, curl up and bring your knees towards your forehead by pulling the legs with your hands. Maintain the position for 10-20 seconds, relax.

○○○

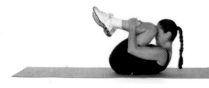

2

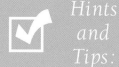

Hints and Tips:

· *Keep your abdominals contracted during the whole exercise.*
· *Focus on the exercise.*
· *If unable to perform this exercise due to pain or fatigue, drop to a lower level or reduce the number of repetitions.*

The One Hundred Series

1 - Initial Position

Lie down on the floor and keep the shoulders relaxed. Maintain the palms of your hands flat against the mat.

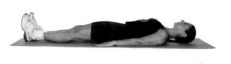

2 - Basic

Bend your knees, maintain the soles of your feet on the mat, lift the shoulders from the floor, and keep the abdominal muscles continuously contracted. Lift your hands from the mat with the palms still facing down and keep your arms straight. Raise your hands up a couple of inches and push them down hard. Perform this motion rhythmically for one hundred arm movements, about twice every second. It's easier if you imagine that you're repeatedly tapping on an invisible pillow, while never touching the mat. Remember to keep the small of your back against the floor.

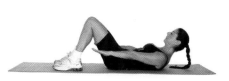

When breathing, exhale slowly through pursed lips, count five arm movements, and inhale. If you're doing the exercise correctly, you'll notice that every time you push the hands down, the contraction of the muscles helps push the air out.

3 - Foot Rest

Same as pose 2, but more difficult. Instead of bending your knees, keep them straight, and rest the heel of one foot over the toes of the other foot.

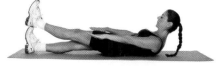

4 - Elevated Legs, Bent

Spice it up. This time bring your thighs to vertical and bend your knees to 45 degrees while doing the one hundred repetitions.

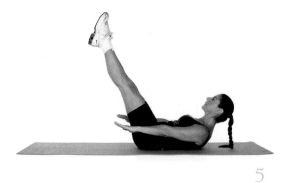

4

5 - Elevated Legs, Straight

Bring the exertion up one more notch by keeping your legs straight and at 45 degrees during the one hundred repetitions.

5

Hints and Tips:

· *Control is the operative word. Perform the exercise slowly and uniformly, without sudden jerks.*
· *Do not pull your neck with your hands.*
· *Twist your shoulder to the opposite side, not your elbows.*

6 - Overhead Reaching

Maximize the exercise by reaching up with your arms once after every ten of the one hundred repetitions; bring the arms straight up from the sides and back down laterally (like doing a backstroke), and repeat another ten of the one hundred repetitions.

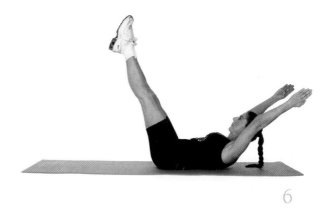

6

7 - Abdominal Bonus Exercise

This exercise engages the oblique abdominal muscles. Start with one leg bent and the other one straight, neither one touching the floor. Bring the shoulder (not the elbow) towards the knee, keeping your hands behind your head. Maintain the abdominals contracted and your shoulders off the mat at all times. Alternate the motion 10-20 times to each side.

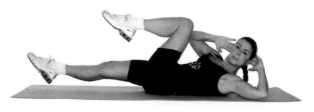

7

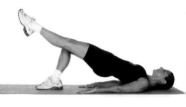

Bridge exercises primarily target the abdominals and the gluteus, and secondarily the arms and legs muscles. They add great strength to the core and they are a fantastic approach to a perfect posture.

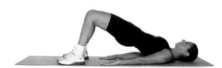

The variation we chose as the best bridge is the Raised Leg Lift, pictured on the opposite page (and pose 8 on page 60), which demands the most from your core, calling for a high level of power, balance, and effort. It's one of a few select exercises that engage such a diversity of muscles.

Remember: Each exercise is labeled with its difficulty level. Be sure to start with Beginner exercises and build your way to Advanced!

●○○	●●○	●●●
Beginner	Medium	Advanced

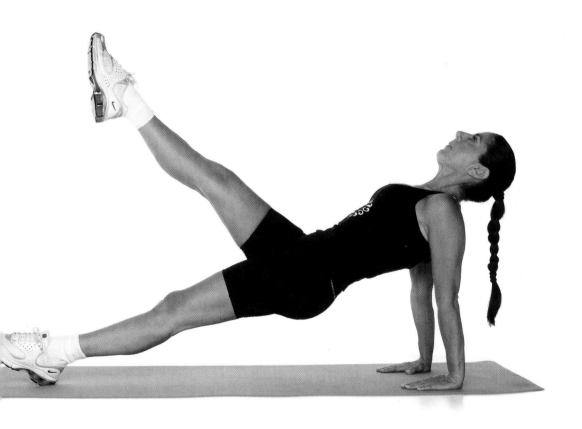

Lower and Upper Stretches

1 - Unilateral Raised Leg

While lying on the floor, reach and hold the leg just below the knee. Maintain position for 10-20 seconds. Release and switch.

●●○

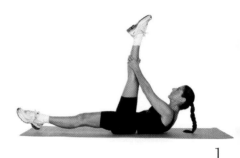

1

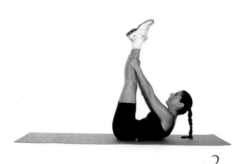

2

2 - Bilateral Raised Leg

Same as stretch 1, this time holding both legs. Maintain position for 10-20 seconds and release.

●●○

3 - Shoulder/Pelvis Stretches

Do this stretch before moving on to the next chapter. Lying face down, stretch your arms out and lower your pelvis until you're sitting on your heels. Hold for 10-20 seconds and release.

●○○

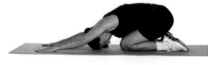

3

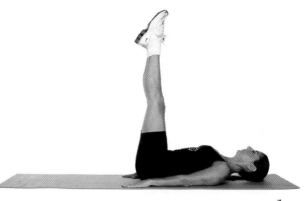

1

1 - Hip Elevations

Before you proceed to the bridge routine, start with a simpler exercise. Keep your legs straight, and lift them up to 90 degrees while keeping the buttocks on the mat.

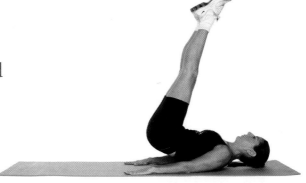

2

2 - Hip Elevations continued

Proceed to raise the buttocks off the mat as if you were trying to reach the ceiling with your feet. Resume the start position and repeat the exercise 10-20 times.

3 - Simple Bridges

Start with your back and arms flat on the mat, knees bent and feet planted on the floor.

●●○

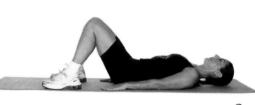

3

4 - Simple Bridges continued

Proceed to slowly raise your hips until your trunk and thighs are aligned. Contract the abs and butt for 1-2 seconds, just enough to lift your hips a couple of inches further; relax without changing your stance. Repeat 10-20 times.

●●○

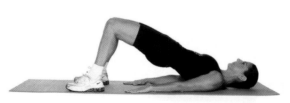

4

5 - Leg Lifts

Make it more difficult by raising one leg up until it's aligned with your thigh and trunk. Contract the abs and butt for 1-2 seconds, just enough to lift your hips a couple of inches further; relax without changing your stance. Repeat 5-10 times each side.

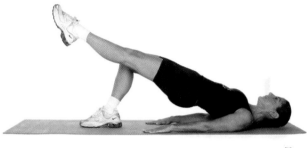

5

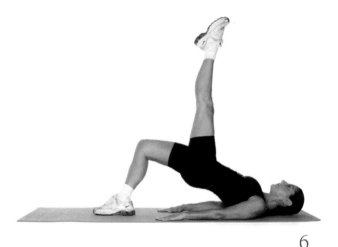

6

6 - Vertical Leg Lifts

Move it up to the highest level of difficulty by raising one leg up until it's vertical. Contract the abs and butt for 1-2 seconds, just enough to lift your hips a couple of inches further; relax without changing your stance. It's easier if you imagine you're reaching to the ceiling with your foot. Repeat 5-10 times each side.

7 - Raised Bridges with Leg Lift

Start with both hands on the floor, arms vertical, and supporting your body in an oblique posture. Contract the abdominals to raise your hips.

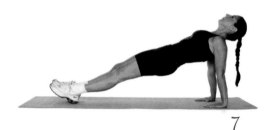

7

8 - Raised Bridges with Leg Lift continued

Proceed to slowly raise one leg to 45 degrees or better. Contract the abs and butt for 1-2 seconds, just enough to lift your hips a couple of inches further; relax without changing your stance. Repeat 5-10 times each side.

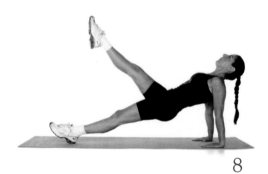

8

Hints and Tips:

·Keep your spine in a neutral position; do not arch your back. Contracting the abs helps.
·Control is the operative word. Perform the exercise slowly and uniformly, without sudden jerks.

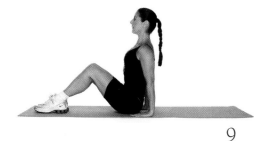

9

9 - Bridges on all Fours

Start seated on the mat, knees bent, hands and feet planted on the floor.

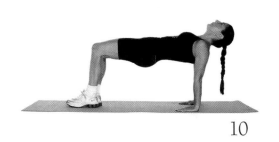

10

10 - Bridges on all Fours continued

Proceed to slowly raise your hips to the ceiling until your trunk and thighs are aligned. Contract the abs and butt for 1-2 seconds, just enough to lift your hips a couple of inches further; relax without changing your stance. Repeat 5-10 times.

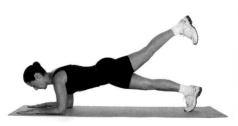

Planks are classic isometric exercises, not relying on continuous movement but instead demanding that the body maintains a certain position for an extended period of time. They don't stress the joints as much as other exercises, but they still provide a great workout.

If you find that the next few exercises are too difficult, move on to the red ball exercise series starting on page 99.

The plank variation we chose as the best, the Straight Alternating Raise, pictured on the opposite page (and pose 12 on page 67), is

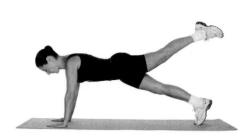

also one of the most difficult to master. To balance the body in such an odd position requires a substantial activation of the trunk muscles and a continuously fine-tuned cooperation among different muscle groups.

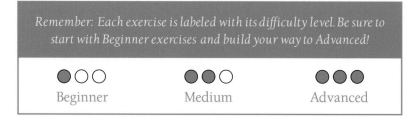

Remember: Each exercise is labeled with its difficulty level. Be sure to start with Beginner exercises and build your way to Advanced!

●○○   ●●○   ●●●
Beginner   Medium   Advanced

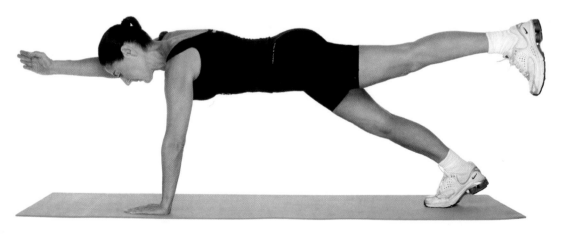

1 - Basic Plank

Start face down, trunk straight, supporting the weight of the body on your elbows and toes. Hold this position for 15-30 seconds.

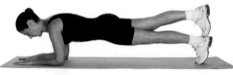

1

2 - Tripod Plank

Same as above but spice it up by resting the toes of one foot over the heel of the other foot.

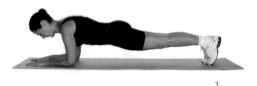

2

3 - Leg Lift Plank

Bring it up one notch by raising one leg straight behind you to 45 degrees. Hold for 15-30 seconds and switch.

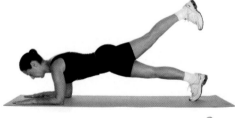

3

Hints · Keep your abdominals contracted during the whole exercise.
and · Pull your navel in toward the spine and rotate the pelvis forward.
Tips: · If you feel unsteady during the exercise, drop to a lower level.

4 - Sideway Swipe Plank

Power it up by moving one leg out to the side while keeping your trunk still. Return to the initial position and switch to the other leg. Repeat 10-20 times each side.

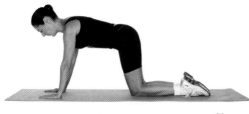

4

5

5 - Extended Plank, Basic

Start on your hands and knees, back straight. Notice that in the next few exercises the center of gravity moves up, making them much more difficult to execute.

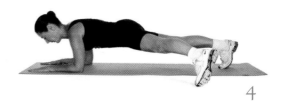

6 - Extended Plank, Basic continued

Proceed to raise your knees up slowly by straightening your legs until they are aligned with your trunk. Keep the abs and butt contracted, and hold this position for 15-30 seconds.

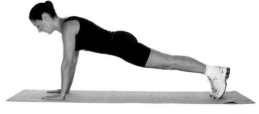

6

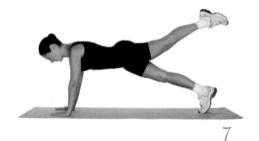

7 - Straight Leg Raise

Spice it up by slowly lifting one leg straight backwards, while raising your hips until your trunk remains horizontal. Hold this position for 15-30 seconds.

7

8 - Bent Leg Raise

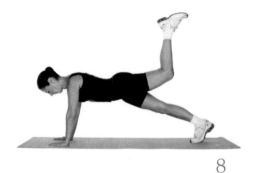

Maximize it by bending the leg at the knee 90 degrees and pushing the foot rhythmically towards the ceiling. Be careful not to overarch your back. Repeat 10-20 times each side.

8

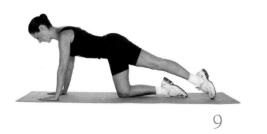

9

9 - Kneeling Alternating Raise

Try this exercise before moving on to an advanced level, acquiring the balance needed to execute more difficult exercises. Start on your hands and knees. Straighten one leg all the way back, still on the floor.

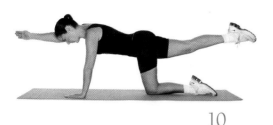

10

10 - Kneeling Alternating Raise continued

Proceed to slowly lift one arm and the opposite leg until they are parallel to the ground. You may choose to lift only one limb at a time, for balance. Maintain the position for 15-30 seconds and switch.

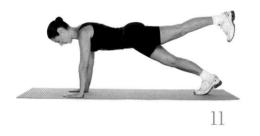

11

11 - Straight Alternating Raise

Start with both hands on the floor and slowly lift one leg straight backwards, while raising your hips until your trunk is horizontal.

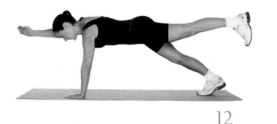

12

12 - Straight Alternating Raise continued

Proceed to slowly lift the hand opposite to the raised leg. Make sure you're stable before you start raising the arm forward until it's parallel to the floor. Maintain the position for 15-30 seconds and switch.

Lumbar Spine Stretche

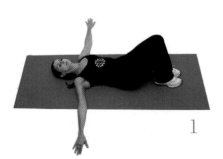

1 - Initial Position

Lie on the floor, arms out to the side and knees bent.

2 - Symmetrical Rotation

Slowly rotate the trunk and place both knees as close to the ground as you can. Hold for 10-20 seconds. Switch sides.

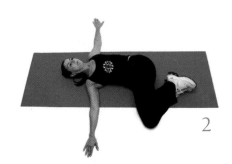

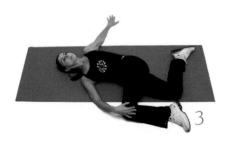

3 - Asymmetrical Rotation

Slowly rotate the trunk and throw the top leg over the bottom one until both knees touch the floor. Hold for 10-20 seconds. Switch sides.

4 - Straight Leg Raise

Slowly raise one leg straight up, aided by pulling with both hands. Hold for 10-20 seconds. Switch sides.

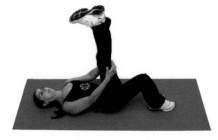

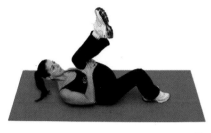

5

5 - Unilateral Knee to Chest

Slowly bring one knee close to the chest, aided by pulling with both hands. Hold for 10-20 seconds. Switch sides.

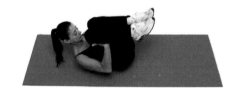

6 - Bilateral Knee to Chest

Slowly bring both knees close to the chest, aided by pulling with both hands. Hold for 10-20 seconds.

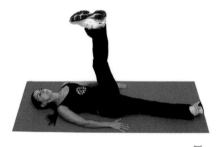

6

7

7 - Straight Leg Rotation

Lie on the floor with both legs straight down. Slowly elevate one leg as close as you can get to 90 degrees.

8 - Straight Leg Rotation continued

Proceed to position one arm out, slowly rotate the trunk and place the foot as close to the ground as you can. Hold for 10-20 seconds. Switch sides.

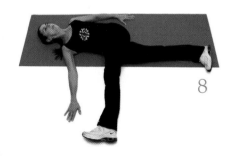

8

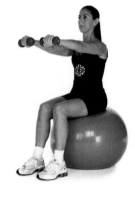

The Swiss ball has become one of the most widely utilized pieces of fitness equipment, and deservedly so for literally hundreds of core exercises have been developed for it. The ball is inexpensive, supple, friendly, and it comes in vibrant colors that invite exercising.

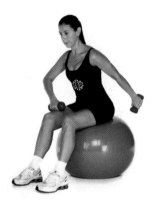

Don't let its playful character fool you since, same as the Swiss ball makes some exercises easier, it makes others devilishly more difficult. Because the ball rolls, most exercises done on it require extra power and further core action to avoid falls during the workout.

Before you advance to the more complex exercises, start with a simpler one, and learn to balance first.

You may choose to do each exercise alone or you may link them together, as an "Around The World" series, adjusting the number of repetitions accordingly.

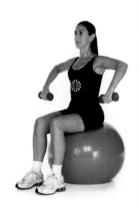

The exercise chosen here as the best variation, the Lateral Arm Raise (pose 6 on page 74), pictured on the opposite page, not only engages the usual core muscles, but it also works the muscles that stabilize the shoulder blades and the neck, necessary for the maintenance of a correct posture.

Remember: Each exercise is labeled with its difficulty level. Be sure to start with Beginner exercises and build your way to Advanced!

●○○	●●○	●●●
Beginner	Medium	Advanced

1 2 3 4 5 6 7 8 9 10

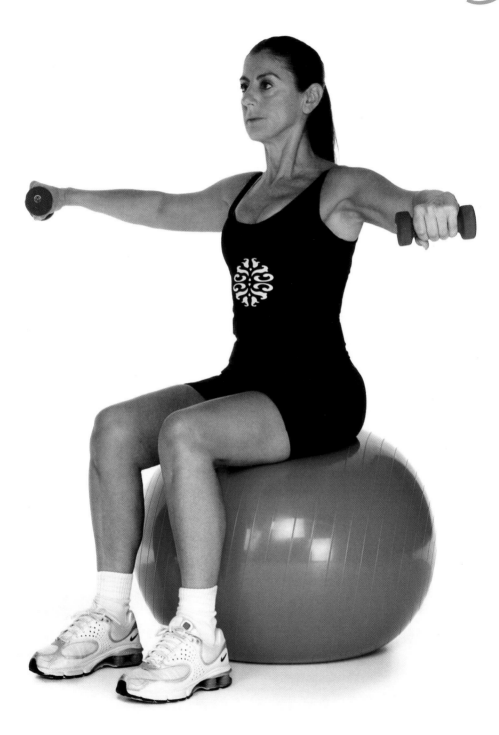

1 - Ball Warm Up, Trunk

If you have never exercised on the ball, try to get the feel for the way it works just sitting on it, moving the pelvis from side to side. After the first few minutes on the ball you'll notice that you're automatically contracting the abdominal and spinal core muscles.

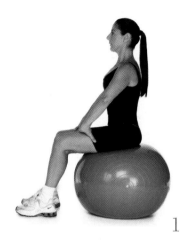

1

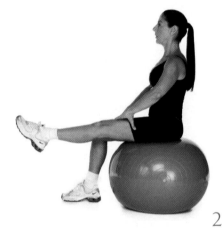

2

2 - Ball Warm Up, Leg

Alternate raising one leg at a time to teach yourself balancing on the ball.

3 - Ball Warm Up, Arms

Proceed to hold your hands behind you. When you feel comfortable with this, spice it up by raising one leg at a time and holding it up for a few seconds.

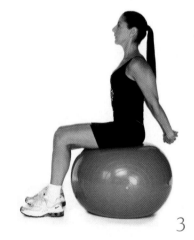

3

Hints and Tips:

· Non-stick mats help stabilize the ball.
· Keep the ball still; don't allow it to roll during the exercise.
· Keep the feet slightly wider than your hips.

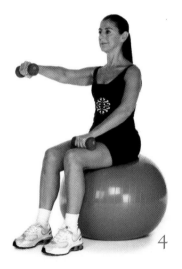

4

4 - Unilateral Forward Raise

Hold a small or medium weight in both hands, resting over the thighs. Raise one arm slowly to shoulder level. Bring it down slowly, while raising the other one. Repeat 10-20 times each side.

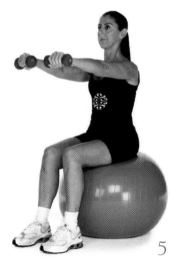

5

5 - Bilateral Forward Raise

When you feel comfortable and secure, try it with both arms simultaneously. Repeat 10-20 times.

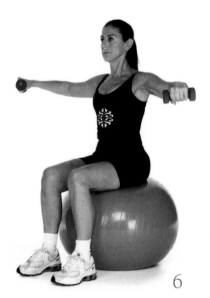

6 - Lateral Arm Raise

Start by holding the weights to your side. Slowly raise your arms and hands out to shoulder level, keeping the elbows slightly flexed. Bring them down slowly. Repeat 10-20 times.

6

7 - Wide Rowing

Start by holding the weights to your side. Slowly raise your elbows to shoulder height while holding the weights down. Resume the initial position. Repeat 10-20 times.

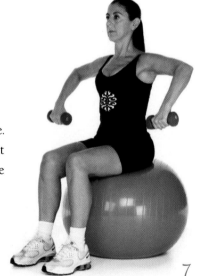

7

8 - Upward Shoulder Rotation

Start by holding the weights over the thighs and raise your elbows to shoulder level and rotate the weights up. Bring them down slowly. Repeat 10-20 times.

●○○

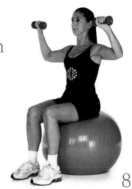

8

9 - Overhead Press

Start by holding the weights over the thighs and raise your arms above the head without locking your elbows. Slowly bring the weights down to shoulder height. Repeat 10-20 times.

●○○

9

10 - Unilateral Triceps Extension

Start by holding one of the weights over your thigh, and slowly move the other arm behind you, keeping your elbow straight. Bring the hand slowly back to your side. Raise it back again, always controlling the movement. Repeat 10-20 times each side.

●○○

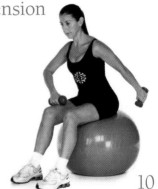

10

11 - Bilateral Triceps Extension

Spice it up by doing the above exercise using both arms simultaneously.

●○○

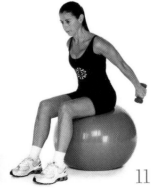

11

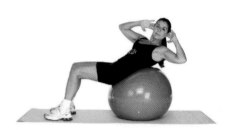

This is another great Swiss ball workout for the core muscles and also for strengthening the limbs. It comprises a challenging routine designed to add spice and variation to the other Swiss ball exercises. Here we target primarily the abdominal and gluteus muscles, which are utilized throughout the various exercises.

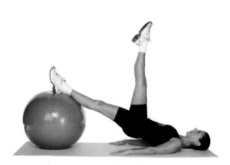

The Vertical Leg Raise variation pictured on the opposite page (and pose 11 on page 81) is our choice as the best posture exercise out of this group. It recruits the core muscles to a very high level because it's a rather unstable position, and only one ankle must prop up a substantial part of the body.

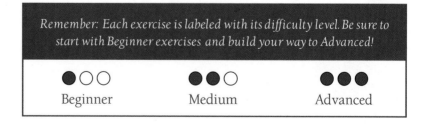

Remember: Each exercise is labeled with its difficulty level. Be sure to start with Beginner exercises and build your way to Advanced!

● ○ ○
Beginner

● ● ○
Medium

● ● ●
Advanced

Ball Exercises for the Abs and Butt 6

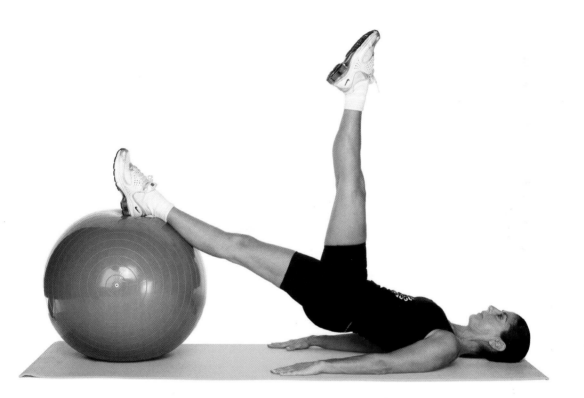

Stretches

Perform the following stretches before changing pace with a new series of exercises. Hold each position for 15-30 seconds.

1 - Trunk Stretch

Start by lying down with the shoulder blades resting on the ball and your feet firmly planted on the ground. Raise your arms above your head.

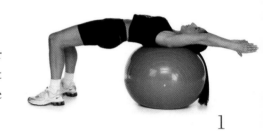

1

2 - Overhead Stretch

Proceed to gradually stretch your legs, allowing the body to relax on the ball.

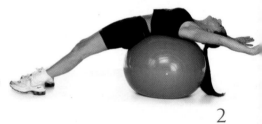

2

3 - Sideways Stretch

Continue by slowly bringing the arms down to your side and let gravity stretch your whole body.

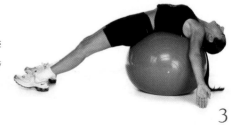

3

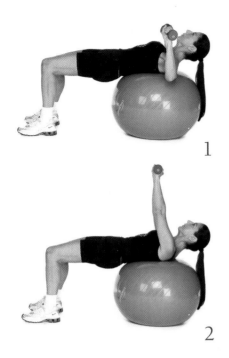

1 - Chest Press

Lie down with the shoulder blades resting on the ball and your feet firmly planted on the ground. Keep the abdominals contracted to maintain the trunk straight. Hold a small to medium size weight in each hand, elbows flexed and pointed out, hands turned up.

2 - Chest Press continued

Proceed to slowly lift the weights toward the ceiling, without locking your elbows. Resume the starting position. Repeat 10-20 times.

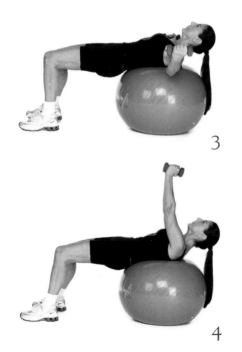

3 - Chest Fly

Start by extending your arms out and to the side, without locking the elbows.

4 - Chest Fly continued

Proceed to slowly bring the arms up and together towards the ceiling. Resume the start position. Repeat 10-20 times.

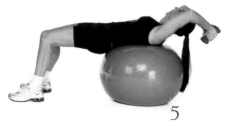

5 - Pullover

Start by holding the weights together, above and behind your head.

● ● ○

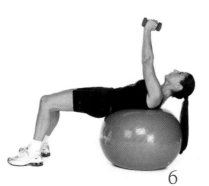

6 - Pullover continued

Proceed to slowly straighten your arms, extending the elbows and pushing the weights toward the ceiling. Resume the start position. Repeat 10-20 times.

● ● ○

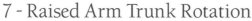

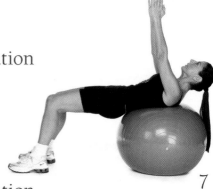

7 - Raised Arm Trunk Rotation

Start by raising your arms up towards the ceiling and hold the palms together.

● ● ○

8 - Raised Arm Trunk Rotation continued

Proceed to slowly rotate your trunk to one side. Hold firmly for three seconds, resume the start position and switch to the other side. Repeat 10-20 times each side.

● ● ○

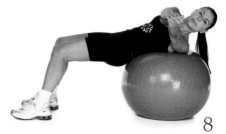

**Hints
and
Tips:**

· If you feel unsteady during the exercise, drop to a lower level.
· Control is the operative word. Perform the exercise slowly
and uniformly, without sudden jerks.

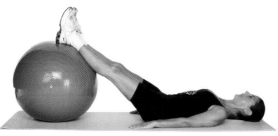

9

9 - Basic Bridge

Lie down on the floor and rest your ankles on the ball. Keep the palms down on the mat.

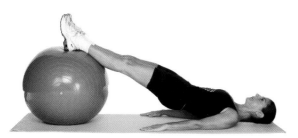

10

10 - Basic Bridge continued

Proceed to slowly raise your hips up until your trunk and thighs are aligned. Contract the abs and butt for 1-2 seconds, just enough to lift your hips a couple of inches further; relax and lower the hips a couple of inches without changing your stance. Repeat 10-20 times.

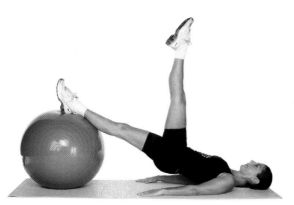

11

11 - Vertical Leg Raise

Bring it up one notch by raising your leg straight to vertical. Contract the abs and butt for 1-2 seconds, just enough to lift your hips a couple of inches further; relax and lower the hips a couple of inches without changing your stance. Repeat 10-20 times each side.

12 - Flexed Knee Bridge

Increase the degree of difficulty another notch. Keep the palms down on the mat. Rest your feet on the ball, raise your hips, but hold the knees semi-flexed. Contract the abs and butt for 1-2 seconds, just enough to lift your hips a couple of inches further; relax and lower the hips a couple of inches without changing your stance. Repeat 10-20 times.

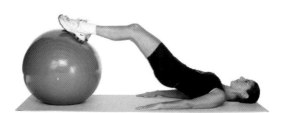

12

13 - Flexed Knee and Vertical Raise

Maximize the exercise by raising one leg up to vertical. Contract the abs and butt for 1-2 seconds, just enough to lift your hips a couple of inches further; relax and lower the hips a couple of inches without changing your stance. Repeat 10-20 times.

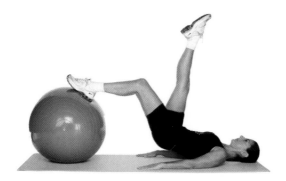

13

Mat Crunches

14 - Lower Abs

Start by lying down, palms on the mat, with your legs at 90 degrees resting on the ball.

15 - Lower Abs continued

Proceed to grab the ball between your ankles and thighs, and bring it towards you. Resume the starting position. Repeat 10-20 times.

16 - Full Abs

Spice it up by lifting the shoulders from the floor towards the knees, feeling the abs contract. Hold the sides of your head with the tips of your fingers. Relax back but don't allow the shoulders to touch the mat. Repeat 15-30 times.

17 - "One Hundred" Abs

Maximize it. Grab the ball with your legs and lift the shoulders from the floor. Always keeping the abdominals engaged, perform the "One Hundred" exercise, as described on page 51.

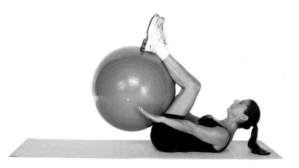

Ball Crunches

18 - Basic

Start by resting on the ball, from the shoulder blades to the lumbar area. Hold the sides of your head with the tips of your fingers. Raise the trunk a few inches, feeling the abdominals contract. Repeat 10-20 times.

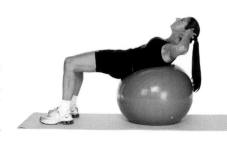

18

19 - Leg Lift

Power it up by doing the abdominal crunches with one leg elevated to 45 degrees. Repeat 10-20 times. Switch legs.

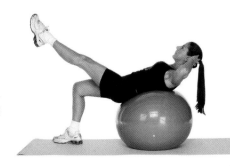

19

20 - Oblique

Engage the abdominal oblique muscles by moving your trunk up and rotating the shoulder to the side. Ease back to the starting position. Repeat 10-20 times each side.

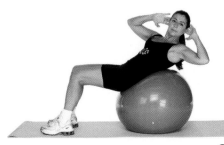

20

Hints and Tips:

· *Stretch slowly. Stay in control.*
· *Keep your abdominals contracted during the whole exercise.*
· *Slowly and surely. Don't let momentum overtake movement.*

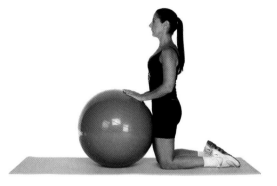

21

Bonus Exercise This

is a great, combined stretch and strengthening exercise for the lateral abdominal muscles.

21 - Kneeling Ball Rotation

Start by kneeling in front of the ball, keep your back straight, and place your hands on the ball.

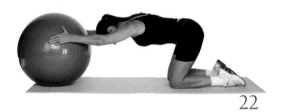

22

22 - Kneeling Ball Rotation continued

Proceed to roll the ball forward, holding it from the sides. Stretch the trunk, keeping it parallel to the ground. Maintain the abdominal muscles contracted.

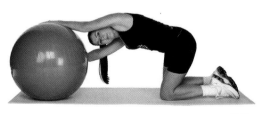

23

23 - Kneeling Ball Rotation continued

Proceed to rotate the ball by twisting your trunk to the side, keeping your knees on the ground. Hold for 3 seconds and resume starting position. Switch to the other side. Repeat 5-10 times each side.

The Plank on the Ball exercises differ from the regular plank routine by freeing the arms. Most of the weight of the upper half of the body in this series rests over the abdomen, adding great leverage to the workout, especially considering that the muscles of the trunk must also support the weight of the arms.

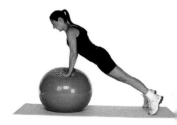

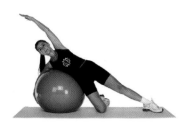

The Superman variation shown on the opposite page (and pose 2 on page 92) is our choice as the best plank on the ball because it activates most of the posterior trunk muscles, enhancing their strength and tone; it is one of the most useful exercises to help you acquire and retain a great posture.

Remember: Each exercise is labeled with its difficulty level. Be sure to start with Beginner exercises and build your way to Advanced!

● ○ ○　　　　● ● ○　　　　● ● ●
Beginner　　　Medium　　　Advanced

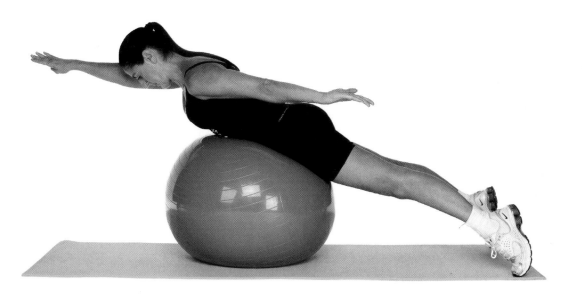

T-Stand

These are active stretching exercises that elongate and tone up the muscles while also working on improving your balance.

1 - Rotated Stretch

Lie face down with the abdomen on the ball, with the hands and the tips of both feet on the floor.

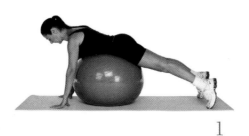

1

2 - Rotated Stretch continued

Proceed to raise one arm up towards the ceiling, twisting your trunk but maintaining both feet on the ground. Hold for 3 seconds and resume the starting position. Switch. Repeat 10-20 times each side.

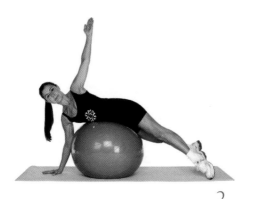

2

**Hints
and
Tips:**

· Keep the feet slightly wider than your hips.
· Do not bend the knees more than 90 degrees.
· Keep the ball still; don't allow it to roll during the exercise.

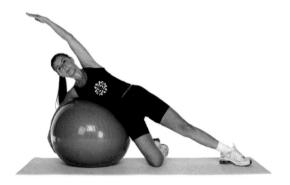

3

3 - Overhead Stretch, Kneeling

Start by kneeling sideways to the ball. Extend the leg farthest away from you and hug the ball with one arm, extending the other up to 45 degrees. Hold for 20-40 seconds. Switch.

●●○

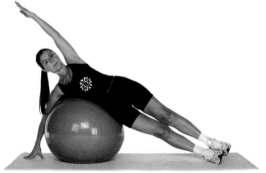

4

4 - Overhead Stretch, Straight

Make it more difficult by extending both legs. Stabilize the position by keeping one hand on the floor and let the trunk muscles do the work. Hold for 20-40 seconds. Switch.

●●○

Kneeling Stretches

Hold each position for 10-20 seconds.

5 - Starting Position

Start by spreading your weight between one foot and one knee. Place your hands on top of the front thigh.

● ○ ○

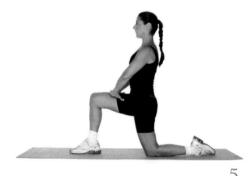

5

6

6 - Quad

Move the front foot forward gradually stretching the posterior leg.

● ○ ○

Hints
and
Tips:

· *Stretch slowly. Stay in control.*
· *Stand tall. Think long.*
· *Keep your ears in line with your shoulders.*

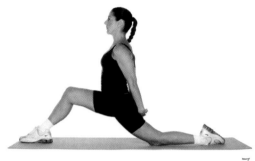

7

7 - Quad / Chest

Move both hands and hold them behind you.

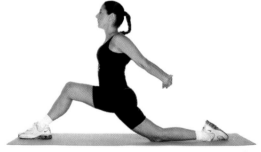

8

8 - Quad / Chest / Arms

Proceed to gradually stretch your arms further back, while keeping the trunk straight.

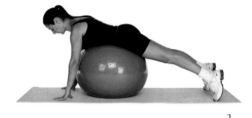

1 - Alternating Arms

Lie face down with the abdomen resting on the ball, with both feet and hands resting on the floor.

1

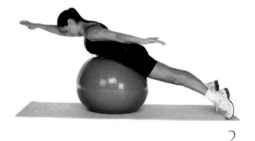

2 - Alternating Arms continued

Proceed to lift one arm forward and the other one backward. Hold for 1-2 seconds and switch to the other side. Repeat 10-20 times each side.

2

Hints and Tips:

· Keep your head neutral, don't force it forward or allow it to drop.
· Avoid excessive tension in the neck.
· Keep your trunk still. Only the limbs perform the exercise.

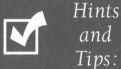

3 - Fingers to Shoulder

Start by resting the abdomen on the ball, with the tip of both feet on the floor, and arms outstretched. Keep your body straight and bend your arms to touch the shoulders with the fingertips. Repeat 10-20 times.

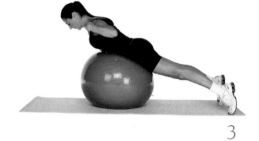

3

4 - Arms Kickback

Spice it up by holding both arms stretched back, parallel to the body. Now push the arms back 2-3 inches while also slightly raising the trunk. Hold for 3 seconds and resume the starting position. Repeat 10-20 times.

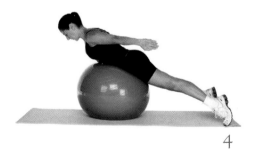

4

5 - Extended Arm Plank

This is a very difficult exercise, demanding an unusual degree of balance and effort. Start by kneeling in front of the ball and placing both hands on it.

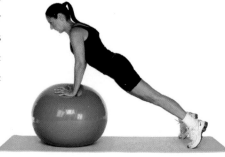

5

6 - Extended Arm Plank
continued

Proceed to slowly straighten the legs out, gradually taking the weight from the knees and distributing it between your hands and feet. Keep your feet and hands apart to enhance stability. Hold the position for 30 seconds. If you feel you're going to fall, quickly bend your knees.

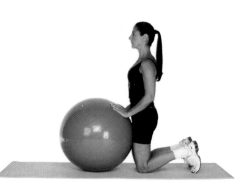

6

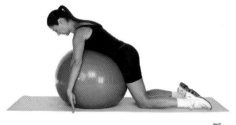

7

7 - Overhead Arm Raise

Start on your knees, resting your abdomen on the ball with your arms hanging down. Keep your back straight.

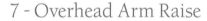

8 - Overhead Arm Raise continued

Proceed to stretch your arms forward, thumbs pointed up. Push the thumbs further up towards the ceiling rhythmically. Repeat 10-20 times.

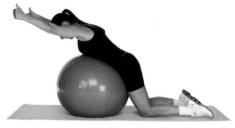

8

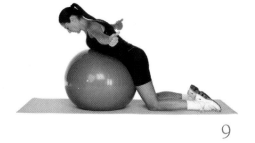

9

9 - Lateral Arm Raise

Add variety by having the thumbs pointed back and up. Push the thumbs further up towards the ceiling rhythmically. Repeat 10-20 times.

10 - Elbows Kickback

Make it a little easier by holding the tips of your fingers to the sides of your head. Push your elbows back and the shoulder blades together rhythmically. Repeat 10-20 times.

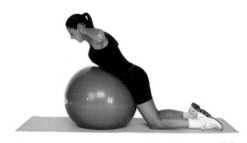

10

Kneeling Weight Lifts

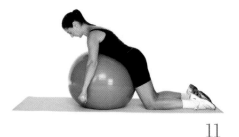

11

11 - Wide Rowing

Start on your knees, resting your abdomen on the ball with your arms hanging down, holding small to medium weights. Keep your back straight.

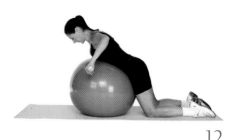

12

12 - Wide Rowing continued

Proceed to raise the weights to chest level, elbows pointed out. Push the elbows back and your shoulder blades together rhythmically. Repeat 10-20 times.

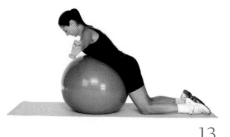

13

13 - Fly

Spice it up, this time with arms stretched out. Push the hand weights up rhythmically. Repeat 10-20 times.

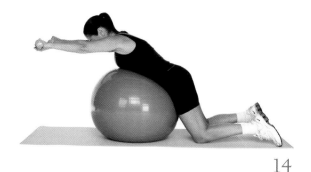

14

14 - Forward Raise

Bring it up one notch by raising the arms forward. Push the hand weights up rhythmically. Repeat 10-20 times.

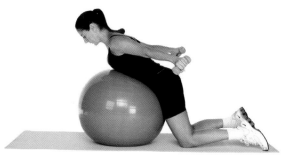

15

15 - Arm Kickback

Make it more difficult by reaching behind you with the weights. Push the hand weights up rhythmically. Repeat 10-20 times.

Straight Leg Weight Lifts

16 - Wide Row

Start with your legs stretched, toes on the floor and resting your abdomen on the ball. Hold small hands weights down on the mat. Keep your back straight.

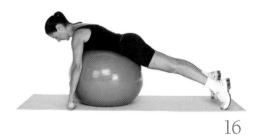

16

●●○

17 - Wide Row continued

Proceed to raise the elbows up. Bring weights up and the shoulder blades together rhythmically. Repeat 10-20 times.

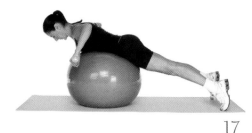

17

●●○

18 - Alternating Arm Raise

Spice it up by alternating each arm forward. Repeat 10-20 times each side.

●●○

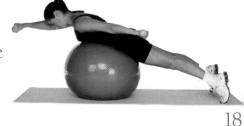

18

19 - Arm Kickback

Make it easier by holding the weights to your side. Push the hand weights up rhythmically. Repeat 10-20 times.

●●○

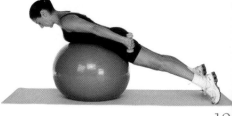

19

Hints and Tips:

·Keep your head neutral, don't force it forward or allow it to drop.
· Avoid excessive tension in the neck.
·If you have trouble stabilizing the ball, rest your feet against the wall to keep it steady.

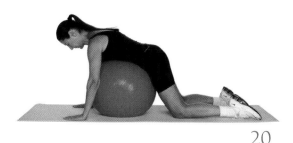

20

Planks on the Ball Variation

20 - Kneeling Arm and Leg Raise

Start on your knees, resting your abdomen on the ball, hands and feet on the floor.

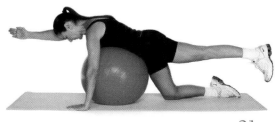

21

21 - Kneeling Arm and Leg Raise continued

Proceed to slowly lift one arm and the opposite leg until they are parallel to the ground. You may choose to lift one limb at a time for balance. Maintain the position for 20-40 seconds and switch.

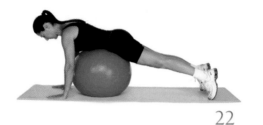

22

22 - Straight Leg Raise

Start by resting the abdomen on the ball with your hands on the mat and both legs straight, feet on the ground.

● ● ○

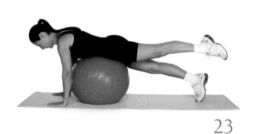

23

23 - Straight Leg Raise continued

Proceed to slowly lift a leg straight backwards, keeping it horizontal. Hold this position for 20-40 seconds.

● ● ○

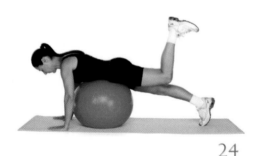

24

24 - Bent Leg Raise

Spice it up by flexing the knee up to 90 degrees and push the foot up rhythmically towards the ceiling. Repeat 10-20 times each side.

● ● ○

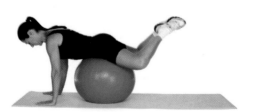

25

25 - Frog Legs

Maximize it by slowly bringing both legs up, and pressing your feet against each other. Keep the abs and butt contracted. Hold the position for 20-40 seconds.

 ● ● ○

Hints
and
Tips:

· *Non-stick mats help stabilize the ball.*
· *Keep the ball still; don't allow it to roll during the exercise.*
· *Focus on the exercise.*

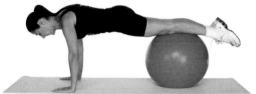

26

26 - Tuck and Pike

Start with the hands on the floor, legs straight over the ball and your trunk parallel to the ground.

27 - Tuck and Pike continued

Proceed to slowly move the ball towards you by bringing the knees close to your chest. Hold the position for 20-40 seconds.

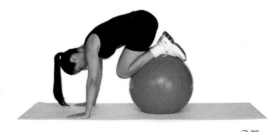

27

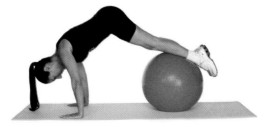

28

28 - Tuck and Pike continued

Proceed to slowly elevate your hips to the ceiling, while straightening your legs out. Hold the position for 20-40 seconds.

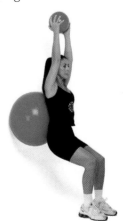

These are exercises that can be done separately or joined together as an Around The World routine, as you build your own customized program. This workout series progresses in the degree of difficulty, engaging more and more of the core muscles as you advance. Like the other examples in this book, it is very important that you try to perform each exercise to perfection every time, in order to obtain the maximum benefit from the program.

The best exercise in this series, the Overhead Raised Leg/Bent knee (pictured on the opposite page and on page 114) is also the most difficult; don't be fooled by how easy it looks in the picture. Most of the weight here is supported by one single leg, bent, while the core muscles must work overtime to stabilize the body. Make sure you've mastered the simpler exercises before trying this one.

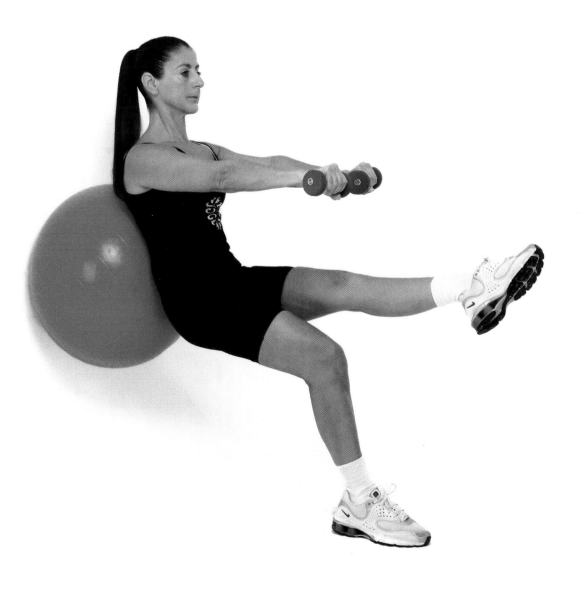

1 - Forward Raise and Twist

Unless noted otherwise, this is the starting position for the next series of exercises. Stand up with your lumbar spine against the Swiss ball, holding your feet slightly apart for stability and a few inches to the front of your hips. If you're not properly balanced you risk getting your body slammed against the wall. Hold a smaller ball low, in front of you. Here we have chosen a light plastic ball but, as you advance, a heavier ball can be utilized.

◓ ◯ ◯

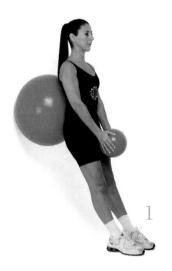

1

2 - Forward Raise and Twist continued

Proceed to raise the ball forward, to shoulder level.

◓ ◯ ◯

3 - Forward Raise and Twist continued

Proceed to rotate your trunk (not your arms) to the side. Slowly begin to get a feel for the exercise. The Swiss ball will rotate some as you move; controlling that rotation is part of what makes this routine so effective for the core muscles. Repeat 10-20 times each side.

◓ ◯ ◯

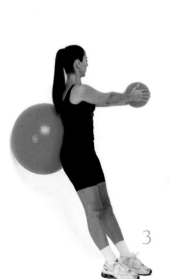

3

4 - Overhead, Bent Knees

Make the routine more difficult by keeping your knees bent to 90 degrees while holding the ball in front of you. If your initial posture against the wall is correct, your knees won't travel further than your ankles.

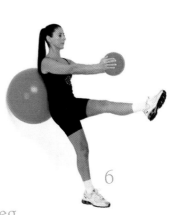

5 - Overhead, Bent Knees continued

Proceed by lifting the ball above your head. Repeat 10-20 times.

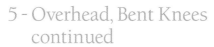

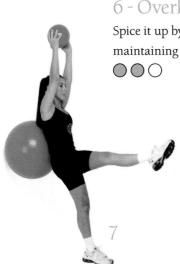

6 - Overhead, Raised Leg

Spice it up by elevating one leg to 90 degrees, maintaining it parallel to the floor.

7 - Overhead, Raised Leg continued

Proceed by lifting the ball above your head. Repeat 10-20 times.

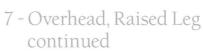

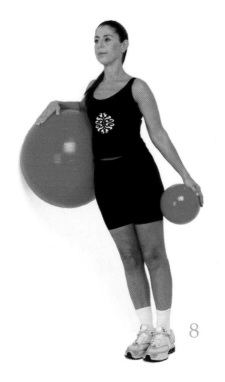

8 - Lateral Overhead

Start by leaning sideways to the ball, resting one arm on top of it and the other one holding the smaller ball to the side.

8

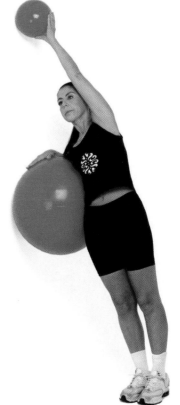

9 - Lateral Overhead continued

Proceed to reach up with the ball until it touches the wall, trying to move further up with each repetition. Resume starting position. Repeat 10-20 times.

9

Hints and Tips:

· *Stand tall. Think long.*
· *Stretch slowly. Stay in control.*
· *Control is the operative word. Perform the exercise slowly and uniformly, without sudden jerks.*

10 - Wall Walking

Start by facing the wall and pressing your abdomen against the Swiss ball. Hold the smaller ball with both hands at chest height.

11 - Wall Walking continued

Proceed to raise your arms up until the ball reaches the wall.

12 - Wall Walking continued

Proceed to move the ball sideways across the wall to one side then to the other. Repeat 10-20 times each side.

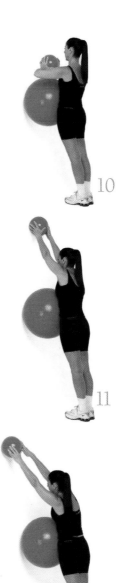

Add Weights

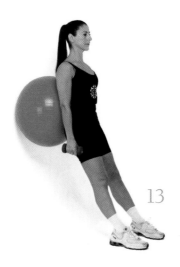

13 - Starting Position

This is the starting position for the next few exercises. Stand up with your lumbar spine against the Swiss ball, in a comfortable fit, and your feet slightly apart for stability. Move the feet a few inches to the front of you hips. Hold a small to medium size weight in each hand, low and to your side.

14 - Curl

Proceed to lift the weights forward to waist level by flexing your elbows to 90 degrees. Resume starting position. Repeat 10-20 times.

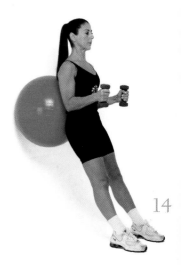

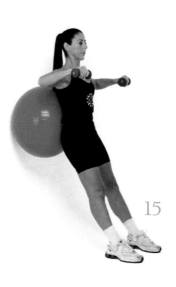

15 - Lateral Raise

Keep the elbows flexed and lift the weights sideways, until they reach shoulder level. Resume starting position. Repeat 10-20 times.

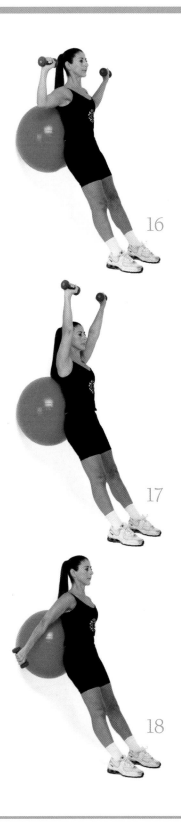

16 - Upward Shoulder Rotation

Lift the weights up to eye level by rotating the shoulders, keeping the elbows flexed. Resume starting position. Repeat 10-20 times.

17 - Overhead Press

Lift the weights up above your head without locking the elbows. Resume starting position. Repeat 10-20 times.

18 - Arm Kickback

Bring the weights behind you and push them back and up rhythmically. Repeat 10-20 times.

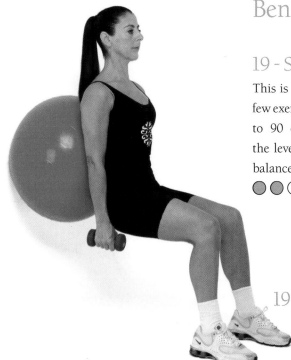

Bent Knees

19 - Starting Position

This is the starting position for the next few exercises. Start with your knees flexed to 90 degrees. This position increases the level of difficulty and requires more balance.

⬤⬤◯

19

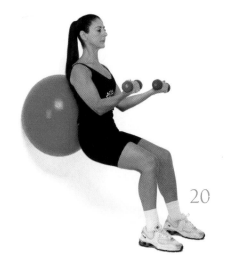

20 - Curl

Lift the weights by flexing your elbows to 90 degrees. Resume starting position. Repeat 10-20 times.

⬤⬤◯

20

Hints and Tips:

· Keep the feet slightly wider than your hips.
· Grip the weights only strong enough to hold them secure.
· Keep your spine in a neutral position; do not arch your back. Contracting the abs helps.

21 - Lateral Raise

Lift the weights sideways, keeping the elbows flexed, until they reach shoulder level. Resume starting position. Repeat 10-20 times.

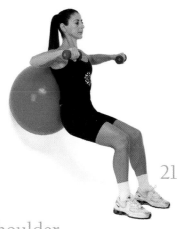

21

22 - Upward Shoulder Rotation

Lift the weights up to eye level by rotating the shoulders, keeping the elbows flexed. Resume starting position. Repeat 10-20 times.

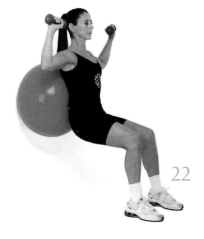

22

23 - Overhead Press

Lift the weights up above your head, without locking the elbows. Resume starting position. Repeat 10-20 times.

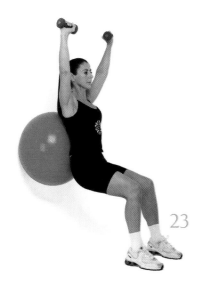

23

Raised Leg

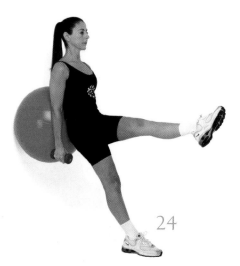

24 - Starting Position

This is the starting position for the next few exercises. It is made more difficult than the preceding exercise by lifting one leg until it's parallel to the ground, keeping the other straight. Start by holding the weights to your side.

24

25 - Curl

Lift the weights by flexing your elbows to 90 degrees. Resume starting position. Repeat 10-20 times.

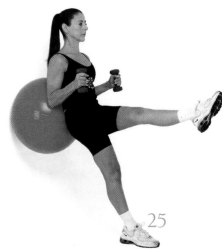

25

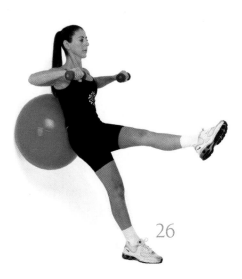

26 - Lateral Raise

Lift the weights sideways, keeping the elbows flexed, until they reach shoulder level. Resume starting position. Repeat 10-20 times.

26

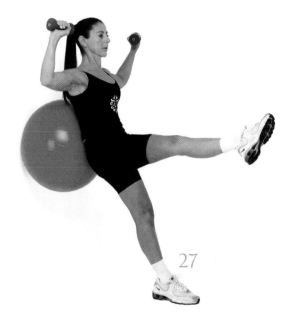

27 - Upward Shoulder Rotation

Lift the weights up to eye level by rotating the shoulders, keeping the elbows flexed. Resume starting position. Repeat 10-20 times.

27

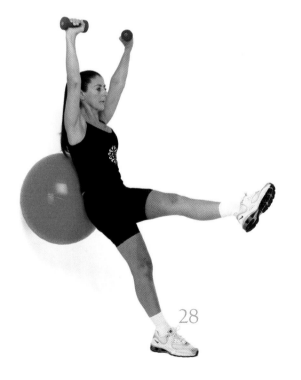

28 - Overhead Press

Lift the weights up above your head without locking the elbows. Resume starting position. Repeat 10-20 times.

28

Raised Leg with Bent Knee

The exercises shown here are an example of an "Around The World" workout, which can be used for the preceding routines also. The exercises are linked together, moving straight from one arm variation to the next one without stopping, keeping the position of the legs unchanged, repeating the arm movements from start to finish. Repeat 10-20 times with each leg.

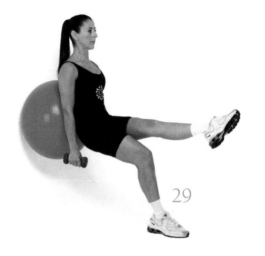

29 - Raise, Pull, Lift

This is the starting position for the next few exercises. Maximize it by lifting one leg until it's parallel to the ground, and flex the other knee to 90 degrees. Begin by holding the weights to your side.

⬤ ⬤ ⬤

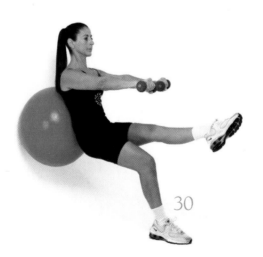

30 - Raise, Pull, Lift continued

Lift the weights straight to shoulder height elevating your arms.

⬤ ⬤ ⬤

Hints and Tips:

· *Inhale and raise the buttocks. Press the foot hard on the floor.*
· *If unable to perform this exercise due to pain or fatigue, drop to a lower level or reduce the number of repetitions.*

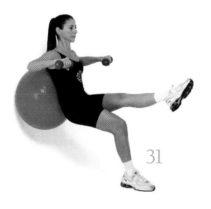

31 - Raise, Pull, Lift continued

Proceed to bring the weights towards your chest by pulling the elbows back.

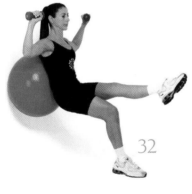

32 - Raise, Pull, Lift continued

Proceed to lift the weights up to eye level by rotating the shoulders, keeping the elbows flexed.

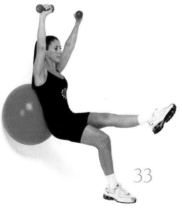

33 - Raise, Pull, Lift continued

Proceed to lift the weights up above your head, without locking the elbows. Resume starting position. Repeat the whole series 10-20 times before changing to the other leg.

W̶e have created Posture², a series of exercises that makes use of a doorframe to help you develop and retain good posture. The doorframe works as a reference, a visual and tactile guide to increase body awareness.

You can also use the doorframe as a clue to remind you of your posture goals. I often stop for a few seconds during my chores to perform one or two of these exercises, just to help me realign my back during the day.

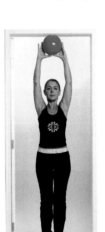

The doorframe exercises work well for people my size. Taller people may need to modify some of these exercises, reaching outside the frame for example, or they may need to find a bigger, non-standard door.

Our favorite workout on this series, the Overhead Slide, pictured on the opposite page (and pose 13 on page 123), stretches the trunk and the limbs as high as they will go, simultaneously strengthening the trunk muscles and solidifying what you have accomplished with the previous routines.

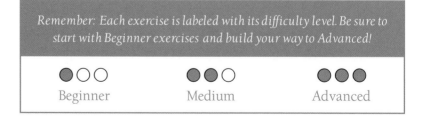

Remember: Each exercise is labeled with its difficulty level. Be sure to start with Beginner exercises and build your way to Advanced!

● ○ ○   ● ● ○   ● ● ●
Beginner   Medium   Advanced

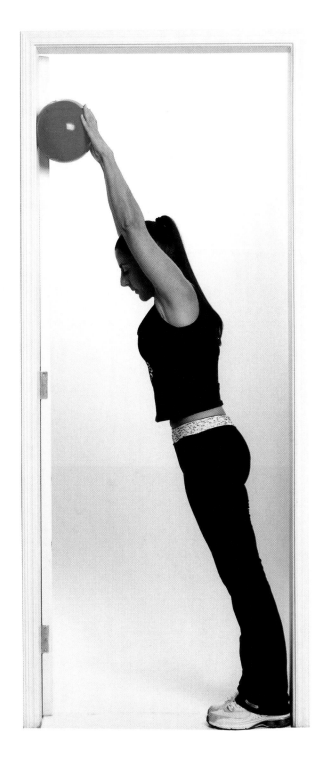

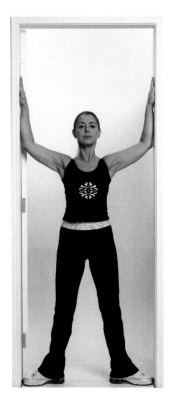

1

1 - Sky Reach

Start feet and arms apart against the doorframe.

●○○

2 - Sky Reach continued

Proceed to slide your arms up towards the top of the frame, standing on your toes, reaching as high as you can, feeling your spine stretch. Resume starting position. Repeat 10-20 times.

●○○

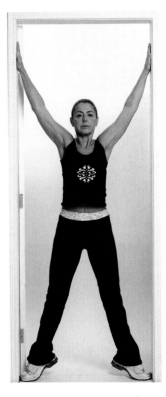

2

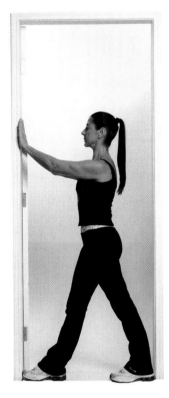

3

3 - Sky Slide

Start with the body sideways, arms touching the frame in front of you and one foot against each wall.

●○○

4 - Sky Slide continued

Proceed to slide both arms up, as high as you can. Notice that the trunk remains straight, without overarching the back. Resume starting position. Repeat 10-20 times.

●○○

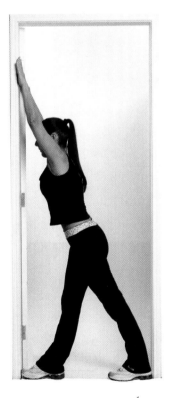

4

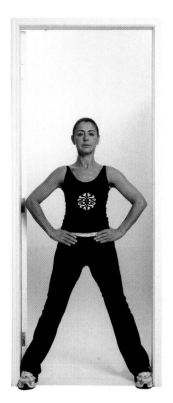

5

5 - Oblique Sky Reach

Start with the sides of your feet against the doorframe, hands on your waist.

● ○ ○

6 - Oblique Sky Reach
continued

Proceed to reach with one hand for the opposite wall and the other hand for the hip. Resume starting position. Repeat 10-20 times each side.

● ○ ○

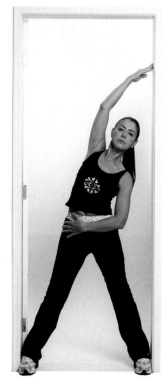

6

*Hints
and
Tips:*

· *Stand tall. Think long.*
· *Stretch slowly. Stay in control.*
· *Keep your spine in a neutral position; do not arch
  your back. Contracting the abs helps.*

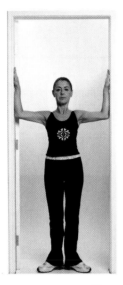

7

7 - Lateral Knee Lift

Start with feet together but toes pointed out
45 degrees, arms against the doorframe.

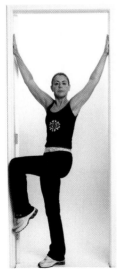

8

8 - Lateral Knee Lift
continued

Proceed to slide your arms up as high as you
can and raise one knee to the opposite side.
Repeat 10-20 times each side.

9 - Straight Knee Lift

Start with your back against the frame, holding it behind you with both hands.

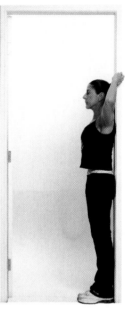

9

10 - Straight Knee Lift
continued

Proceed to slide the hands up, reaching as high as you can, while raising one knee until the thigh is parallel to the floor. Resume starting position. Repeat 10-20 times each side.

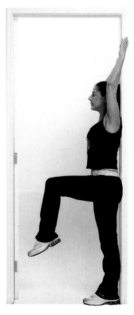

10

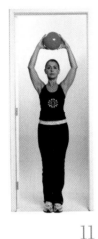

11

11 - Overhead Reach

Start by standing up at the center of the doorframe. Hold a ball with both hands above your head, elbows semi-flexed.

● ○ ○

12 - Overhead Reach continued

Proceed to reach up to the top of the doorframe, or behind it if you're tall enough. Repeat 10-20 times.

● ○ ○

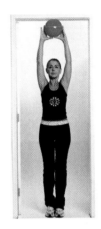

12

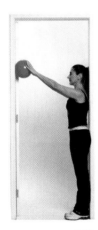

13

13 - Overhead Slide

Start by leaning your back against the doorframe. Hold a ball with both arms and reach forward.

● ● ○

14 - Overhead Slide continued

Proceed to slowly roll the ball up against the frame as high as you can. Be careful not to overarch the back. Hold for 20-40 seconds.

● ● ○

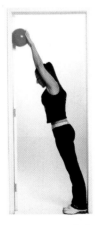

14

E lastic bands have been mistaken as toys or as providing a lesser quality of exercise. In fact, some of the best exercises for the muscles of the trunk involve the use of elastic bands or tubes. Elastic bands come in many different resistances, so they can accommodate a variety of people, from beginners to pros. They are great for those on the move who may carry with them just one or two different bands to attain a wide range of exercises; just fold one band in two and you have immediately doubled its resistance. Neat.

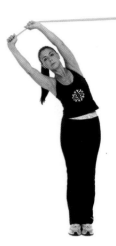

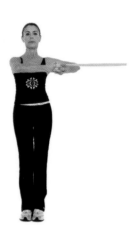

For this fitness routine I recommend placing three solid hooks on a wall at different heights. Locate the high one a few inches above your head, the middle one at shoulder level, and the lower one at knee height. An iron gate or a fence constitutes a reasonable alternative to place the bands; just make sure it's a solid connection. *Warning: elastic bands do hurt if they come loose, and they can cause serious injury if not properly secured.*

Although it appears redundant, repeating the exercises from all three different heights works on distinct muscle groups.

The exercise pictured on the opposite page, the Rotated Outward Pull (also on page 134) is my favorite one in this series, simple and straightforward, but very effective. It opens the chest, stabilizes the shoulder blades, and increases posture awareness.

Remember: Each exercise is labeled with its difficulty level. Be sure to start with Beginner exercises and build your way to Advanced!

●○○   ●●○   ●●●
Beginner   Medium   Advanced

Elastic Bands 10

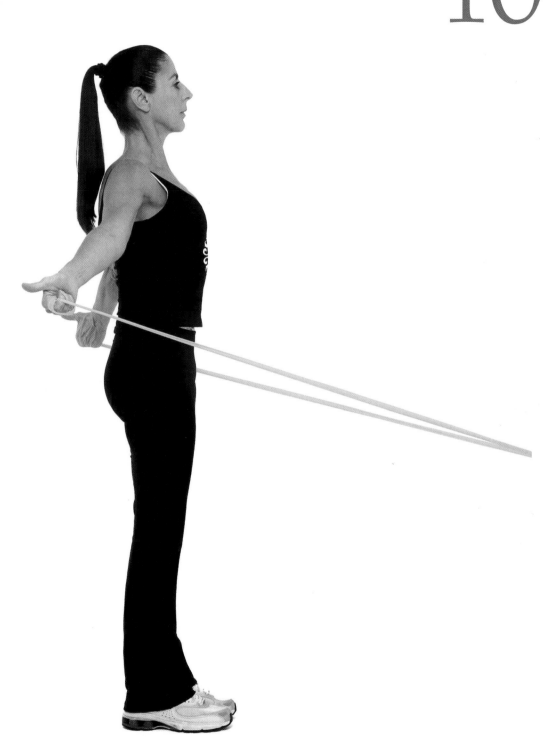

Upper Band Position

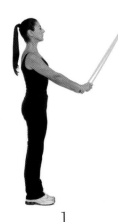

1

1 - Lateral Pull, Low

Start at the top level facing forward and holding equal lengths of the band. Pull them down in front of you with arms straight until you feel some resistance.

●○○

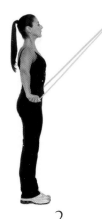

2 - Lateral Pull, Low continued

Proceed to pull the bands down and to your side, a few inches from the body. Resume the starting position. Repeat 10-20 times.

●○○

2

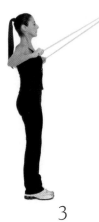

3

3 - Lateral Pull, High

Start by pulling the bands towards you, until your hands get close to your chest.

●○○

4 - Lateral Pull, High continued

Proceed to pull the bands out and to your side. at shoulder height. Resume the starting position. Repeat 10-20 times.

●○○

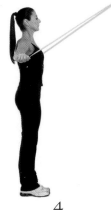

4

Hints and Tips:

· Stand tall. Think long.
· Keep your ears in line with your shoulders.
· Slowly and surely. Don't let momentum overtake movement.

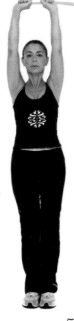

5 - Sideways Pull

Start by standing sideways to the wall, holding the bands above your head, arms straight.

5

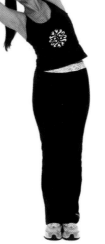

6 - Sideways Pull continued

Proceed to pull the bands to your side. Resume the starting position. Repeat 10-20 times each side.

6

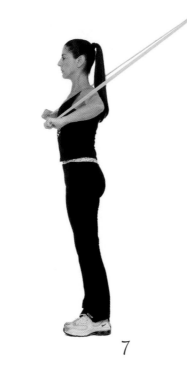

7

7 - Downward Push

Start with your back to the wall, elbows flexed, and hands slightly below chest level.

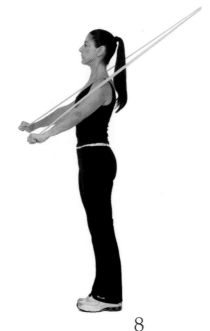

8

8 - Downward Push continued

Proceed to stretch your arms down and out following the same path they were pointed at the beginning, in a smooth motion. Resume the starting position. Repeat 10-20 times.

Hints and Tips:

· Pull your navel in toward the spine and rotate the pelvis forward.
· Stretch slowly. Stay in control.
· Focus on the exercise.

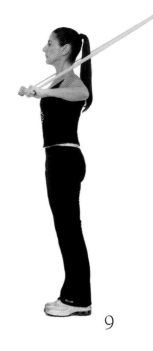

9

9 - Forward Push

Start with your back to the wall, elbows flexed, and hands at chest level.

10 - Forward Push continued

Proceed to stretch your arms out horizontally, in a smooth motion. Resume the starting position. Repeat 10-20 times.

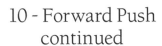

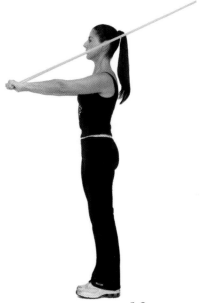

10

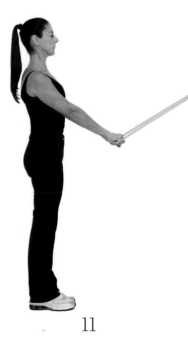

11

Middle Band Position

11 - Lateral Pull, Low

Start with the band at the middle level facing forward and holding equal lengths of the band. Pull them down in front of you with arms straight until you feel some resistance.

● ○ ○

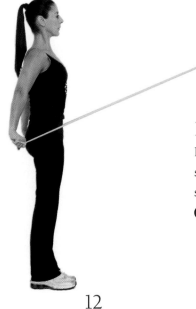

12

12 - Lateral Pull, Low continued

Proceed to pull the bands down and to your side, 45 degrees from the body. Resume the starting position. Repeat 10-20 times.

● ○ ○

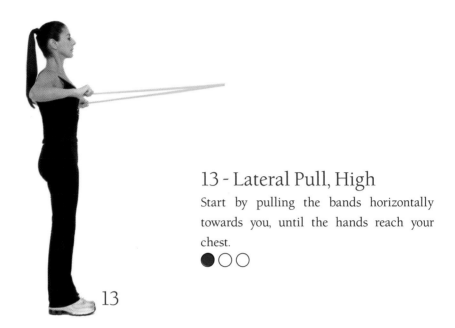

13 - Lateral Pull, High

Start by pulling the bands horizontally towards you, until the hands reach your chest.

●○○

13

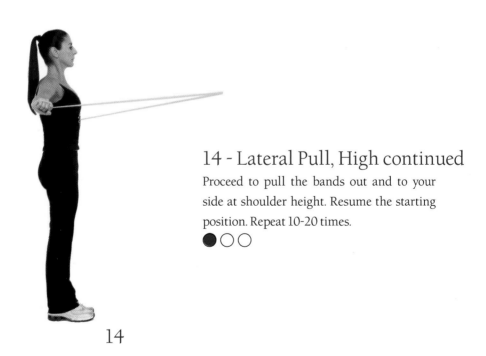

14 - Lateral Pull, High continued

Proceed to pull the bands out and to your side at shoulder height. Resume the starting position. Repeat 10-20 times.

●○○

14

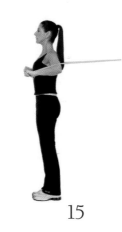

15 - Forward Push

Start facing back to the wall, elbows flexed, and hands at chest level.

●○○

15

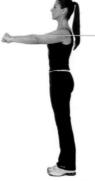

16 - Forward Push continued

Proceed to stretch your arms forward holding them horizontally in a smooth motion. Resume the starting position. Repeat 10-20 times.

●○○

16

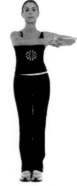

17 - Lateral Twist

Start by standing sideways to the wall holding the bands to your side at chest level.

●○○

17

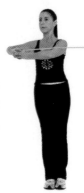

18 - Lateral Twist continued

Proceed to pull the bands to the opposite side, keeping them at chest level. Resume the starting position. Repeat 10-20 times each side.

●○○

18

1
2
3
4
5
6
7
8
9
10

Hints and Tips:

· *Control is the operative word. Perform the exercise slowly and uniformly, without sudden jerks.*
· *Keep your spine in a neutral position; do not arch your back. Contracting the abs helps.*

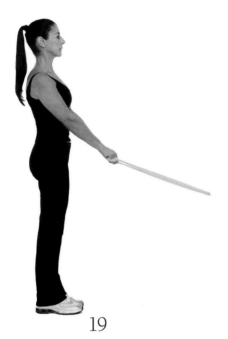

19

Low Band Position

19 - Chest Pull

Start facing forward and holding equal lengths of the bands. Keep your arms straight and shorten the bands until you feel some resistance.

20 - Chest Pull continued

Proceed to pull the bands by flexing your elbows until your hands get to chest height. Resume the starting position. Repeat 10-20 times.

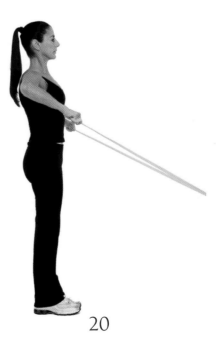

20

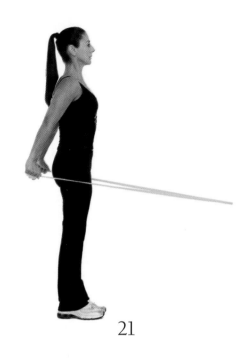

21

21 - Rotated Outward Pull

Start facing forward and holding the bands with arms parallel to the body, hands slightly behind you. Pull until you feel some resistance.

●○○

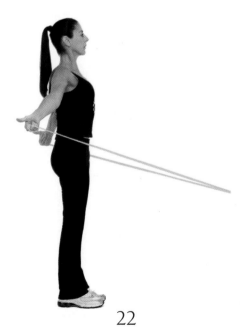

22

22 - Rotated Outward Pull continued

Proceed to pull the bands out and back by rotating your thumbs out and moving your arms 45 degrees away from your body. Resume the starting position. Repeat 10-20 times.

●○○

23 - Side Pull

Start by standing sideways to the wall holding the bands to your side at waist level, using the hand farthest away from the bands.

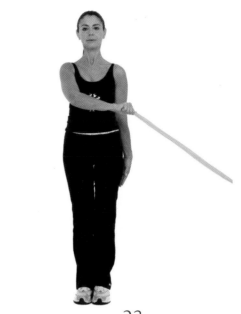

23

24 - Side Pull continued

Proceed to pull the bands sideways and up. Resume the starting position. Repeat 10-20 times each side.

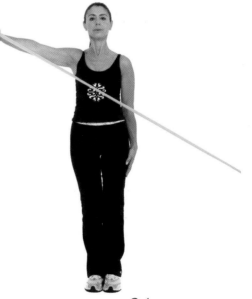

24

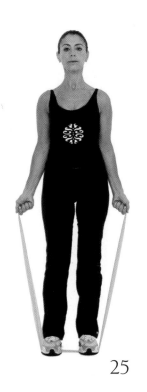

25

No Wall Required
Add these exercises to your routine or do them by themselves anytime you wish, since you can carry these bands wherever you go.

25 - Starting Position

This is the starting position for the next few exercises. You may choose to do them separately or, preferably, you may link them as an "Around The World" routine. Start by standing up with your feet over the middle of the bands. Hold each extremity of the bands with some tension, arms down.

● ○ ○

26 - Curl

Proceed to bring the bands chest high by flexing the elbows. Resume the starting position. Repeat 10-20 times.

● ○ ○

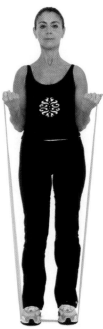

26

Hints and Tips:

· Stand tall. Think long.
· Keep your trunk still. Only the limbs perform the exercise.
· Relax the shoulders by increasing the distance between your shoulders and your ears.

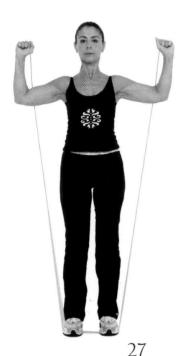

27

27 - Shoulder Rotation

Proceed to bring the bands to your side at eye level, shoulders rotated up. Resume the starting position. Repeat 10-20 times.

●○○

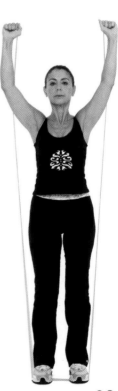

28 - Overhead Press

Proceed to bring the bands above your head by extending the arms up without locking the elbows. Resume the starting position. Repeat 10-20 times.

●○○

28

You've worked hard and you deserve a break. Breathing exercises expand the rib cage, improve posture and, equally as important, they allow the mind to relax. Be careful when standing up after performing these exercises because either dizziness or a drop in blood pressure can occur after deep breathing.

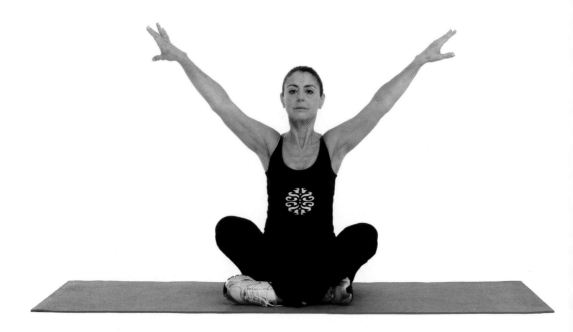

Relaxation Exercises

1

Start seated on the floor with your legs crossed, arms on your lap, palms on top of each other facing up. As you breathe deeply, slowly extend your arms out until they are horizontal, and feel the rib cage muscles stretch. As you exhale, bring the arms slowly back to the initial position. Breathe deeply 5-10 times.

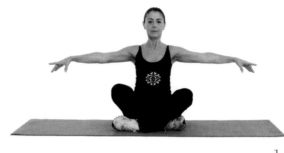

1

2

Bring it up a notch by elevating the arms to 45 degrees while breathing; it stretches the rib cage further. Breathe deeply 5-10 times.

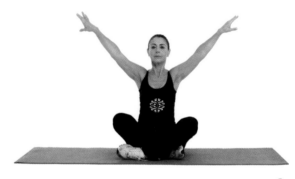

2

3

Add some spice by having one leg crossed in front of you and the other one extended behind you. Breathe deeply 5-10 times each side.

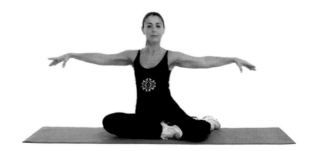

3

E ventually all of us have to slow down, either due to age or illness, but that's no reason to stop working on our posture. We have included some exercises considered as safe alternatives and a good starting program for people who are weak or deconditioned.

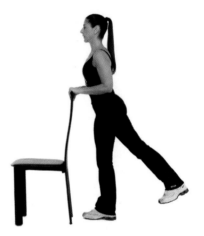

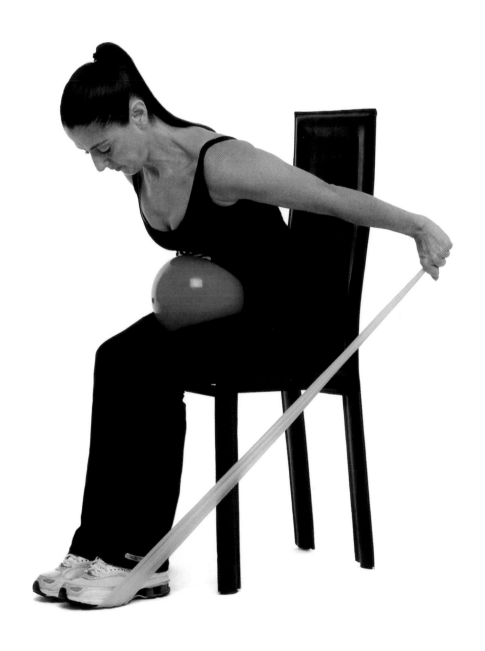

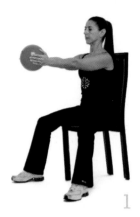

1 - Trunk Rotation

Start seated in a chair with your back supported. Hold a ball with both hands away from you, at chest height.

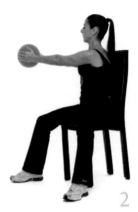

2 - Trunk Rotation
continued

Proceed to rotate the ball utilizing your trunk, not your arms. Resume the starting position. Repeat 5-10 times each side.

3 - Arm Raise

Start as in position 1, but this time raise the ball above your head. Resume the starting position. Repeat 5-10 times.

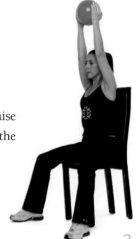

Hints and Tips:
· Try to work at the same speed throughout the exercise.
· The farther the hands are from the trunk, the higher the degree of difficulty.
· Rotate only the upper half of your body by keeping your feet planted on the ground.

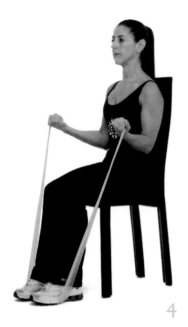

4

4 - Curl

Start seated in a chair with your back supported. Hold the bands with both hands low and to your side. Bring the bands up to chest level by flexing your elbows. Resume the starting position. Repeat 5-10 times.

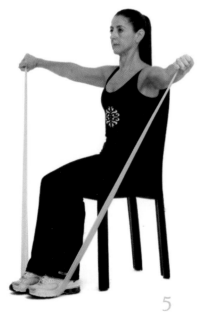

5

5 - Lateral Raise

Hold the bands with both hands low and to your side. Raise the bands up and sideways, extending the arms until they reach shoulder level. Resume the starting position. Repeat 5-10 times.

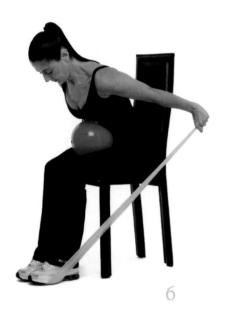

6 - Triceps Extension

Start seated in a chair with your abdomen leaning over and supported by a ball on your lap (this takes pressure off of the spine). Hold the bands with both hands to your side. Proceed to move your arms backwards and up. Resume the starting position. Repeat 5-10 times.

6

7 - Outward Thumb Rotation

Spice it up by pointing the thumbs up and out. Feel the tension between the shoulder blades. Resume the starting position. Repeat 5-10 times.

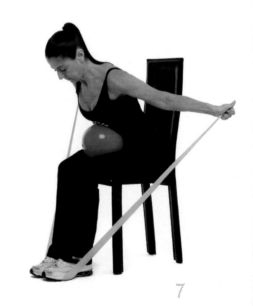

7

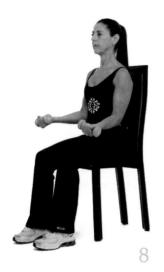

Weights Added

8 - Curl

Start sitting in a chair with your back supported. Hold small weights in both hands, arms parallel to the ground, elbows flexed at 90 degrees.

●○○

8

9 - Curl continued

Proceed to raise the hands up, bringing the weights close to your chest. Resume the starting position. Repeat 5-10 times.

●○○

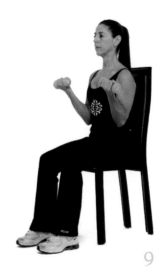

9

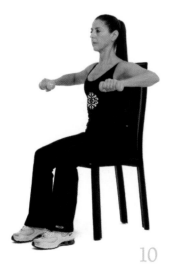

10 - Lateral Raise

This time bring the weights sideways to shoulder height. Resume the starting position. Repeat 5-10 times.

●○○

10

11 - Upward Shoulder Rotation

This time bring the weights up to eye level by rotating the shoulders. Resume the starting position. Repeat 5-10 times.

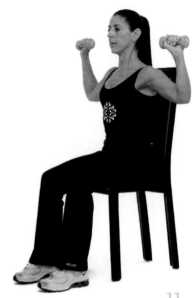

11

12 - Overhead Press

Raise the hands up bringing the weights straight above your head without locking your elbows. Resume the starting position. Repeat 5-10 times.

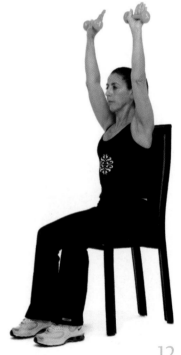

12

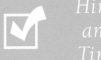

Hints and Tips:

· *Try to work at the same speed throughout the exercise.*
· *Grip the weights only strong enough to hold them secure.*
· *Control is the operative word. Perform the exercise slowly and uniformly, without sudden jerks.*

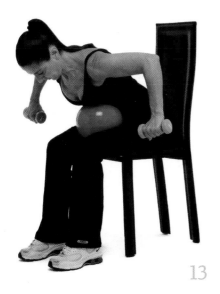

13

13 - Triceps Extension

Start seated in a chair with your abdomen supported by a ball on your lap. Hold the weights in both hands to your side, elbows flexed at 90 degrees.

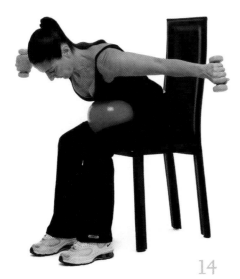

14

14 - Triceps Extension continued

Proceed to raise the weights up to shoulder level and back by extending your arms. Resume the starting position. Repeat 5-10 times.

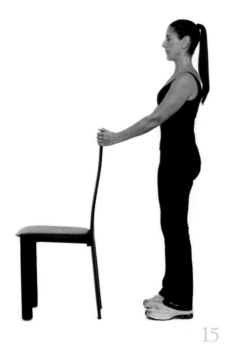

Supported Standing

The next few exercises are aimed at people with restricted mobility and balance. You are encouraged to be creative and to adapt the exercises to any limitations you may have. It's never too late to work on your posture.

15 - Starting Position

Start standing, with both hands to a chair high enough to hold comfortably.

●○○

15

16 - Squat

Proceed to slowly bend your knees to 45 degrees. Hold for 3 seconds. Resume the initial position. Repeat 10-20 times.

●○○

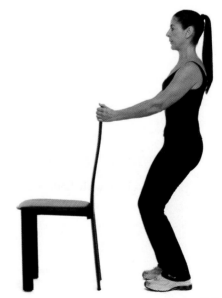

16

17 -Forward Leg Raise

Keep one hand on the chair and the other at the waist. Slowly lift the leg farthest to the chair to 45 degrees. Resume the initial position. Repeat 10-20 times.

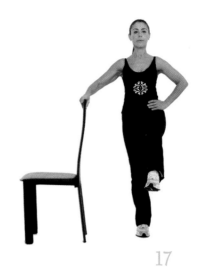

17

18 -Backward Leg Raise

Hold the chair with both hands. Slowly lift one leg back to 45 degrees, knee straight. Resume the initial position. Repeat 10-20 times with each leg.

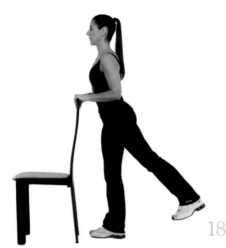

18

19 -Lateral Leg Raise

Hold the chair with both hands, sideways. Slowly lift one leg to the side 45 degrees, knee straight. Resume initial position. Repeat 10-20 times with each leg.

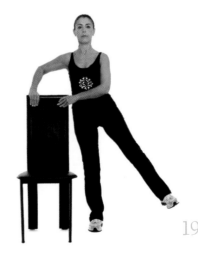

19

I f you feel overwhelmed with the number and variety of exercises and can't make up your mind about which workout combination would be the best for you, don't worry. We selected some of the exercises and grouped them according to their degree of difficulty in three categories: Beginner, Advanced, and Ten-Minute Power Core.

Use these suggestions as a starting point and modify them by subtracting or adding other exercises to make a routine that matches your body and your spirits. You can design different routines for indoors and outdoors, for lazy days and hectic days. Be creative.

Combined Exercise Options

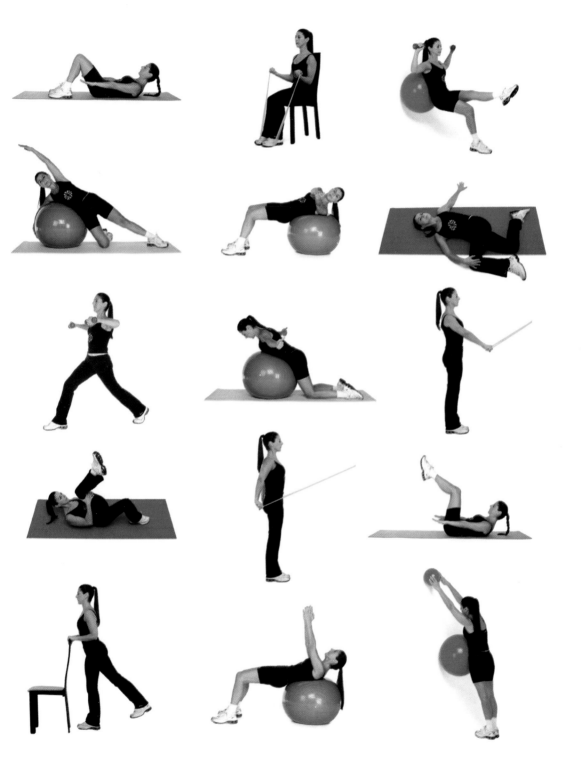

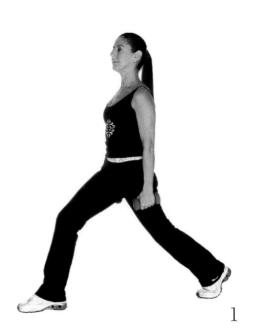

Beginner's Routine

If you consider yourself a novice, start with the following fitness routine. Perform the exercises slowly and carefully. Stop and rest if you feel tired or short of breath. When in doubt, consult your doctor before engaging in any workout.

1 - from page 45-2
5-10 repetitions

1

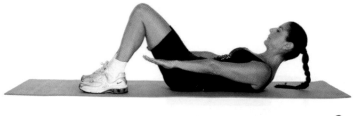

2 - from page 51-2
Cut the "One-Hundred" to
fifty repetitions only

2

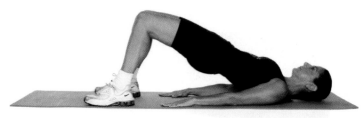

3 - from page 58-4
5-10 repetitions

3

Hints
and
Tips:

· Focus on the exercise.
· Stand tall. Think long.
· Slowly and surely. Don't let momentum overtake movement.

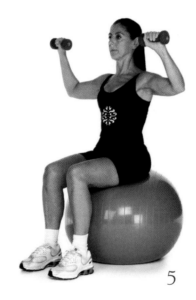

4

4 - from page 64-1
5-10 repetitions

5

5 - from page 75-8
5-10 repetitions

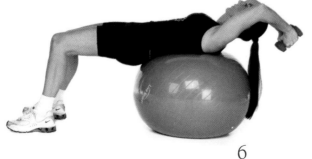

6

6 - from page 80-5
5-10 repetitions

7 - from page 83-15
5-10 repetitions

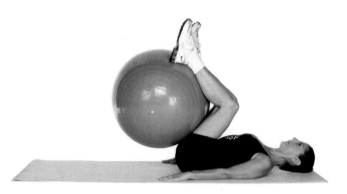

7

8 - from page 95-10
5-10 repetitions

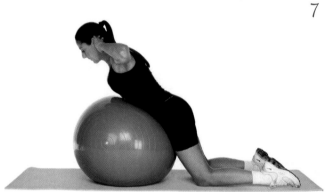

8

9 - page 104-3
5-10 repetitions

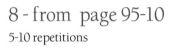

9

10 - from page 118-2
5-10 repetitions

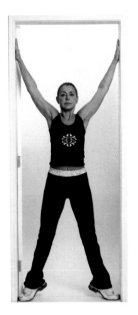

10

11 - from page 126-3
5-10 repetitions

11

12 - from page 137-28
5-10 repetitions

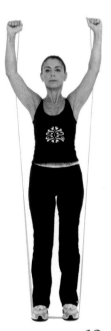

12

Advanced Routine

If you consider yourself a pro, go ahead with the following routine. Be careful because it may be difficult even for those who are experienced. When in doubt, stop and reevaluate what you're doing. Better to be safe than sorry.

1 - from page 47-7
5-10 repetitions with each leg

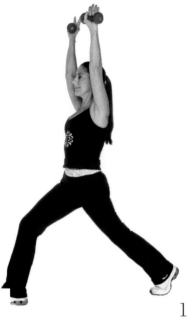

1

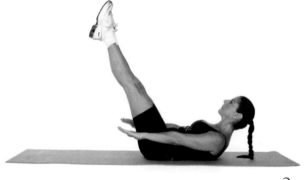

2

2 - from page 52-5
Do the "One-Hundred"

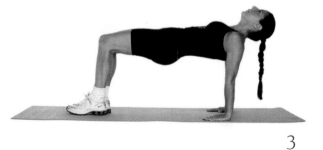

3

3 - from page 61-10
5-10 repetitions

Hints and Tips:
· If you feel unsteady during the exercise, drop to a lower level.
· If unable to perform this exercise due to pain or fatigue, drop to a lower level or reduce the number of repetitions.

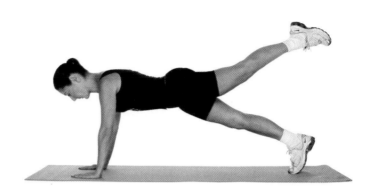

4 - from page 66-7
5-10 repetitions with each leg

4

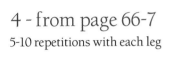

5 - from page 60-8
5-10 repetitions with each leg

5

6 - from page 59-6
5-10 repetitions with each leg

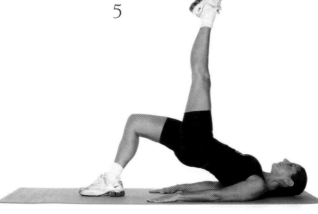

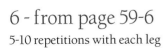

6

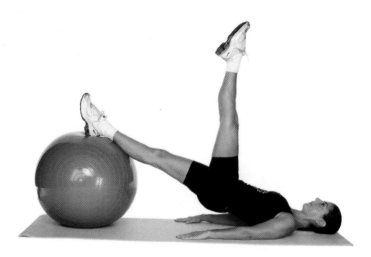

7 - from page 81-11
5-10 repetitions with each leg

7

8 - from page 98-19
5-10 repetitions

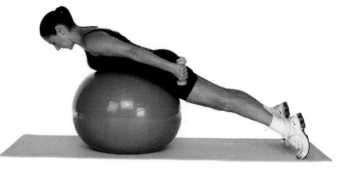

8

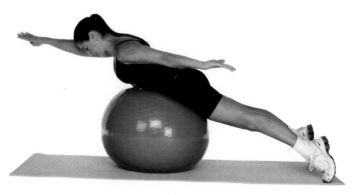

9 - from page 92-2
5-10 repetitions with each arm

9

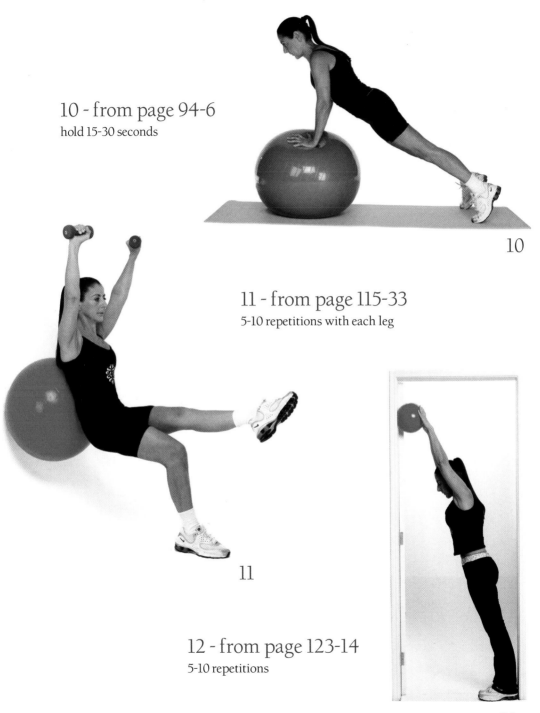

10 - from page 94-6
hold 15-30 seconds

10

11 - from page 115-33
5-10 repetitions with each leg

11

12 - from page 123-14
5-10 repetitions

12

10-Minute Power Core

If you consider yourself an expert but you don't have much time for a workout, try this fitness routine. Perform the exercises slowly and carefully; don't rush through them or you risk getting injured.

1 - from page 53-6
Do the "One Hundred"

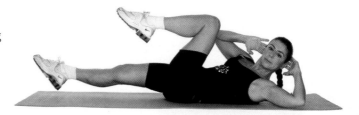

1

2 - from page 53-7
5-10 repetitions with each leg

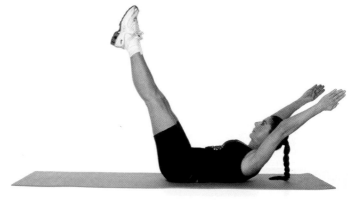

2

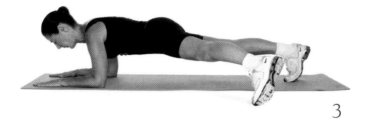

3 - from page 65-4
5-10 repetitions with each leg

3

4 - from page 66-7
5-10 repetitions with each leg

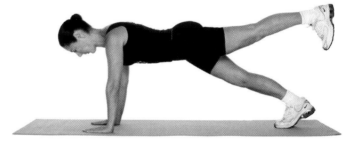

4

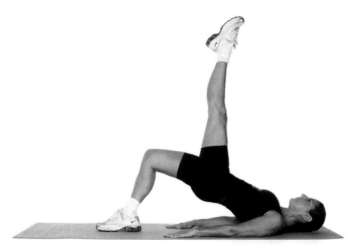

5 - from page 59-6
5-10 repetitions with each leg

5

6 - from page 82-13
5-10 repetitions with each leg

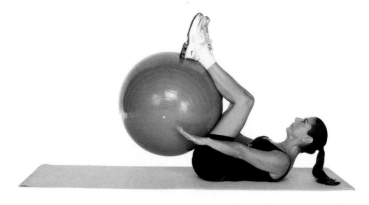

6

7 - from page 83-17
Do the "One Hundred"

7

8 - from page 88-2
5-10 repetitions with each arm

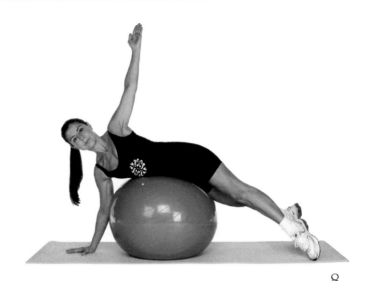

8

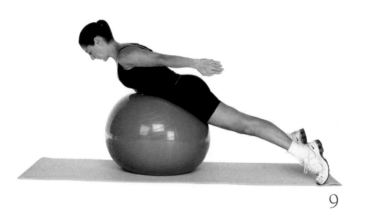

9

9 - from page 93-4
5-10 repetitions

10 - from page 101-26 to 28
Hold each position for 15-30 seconds

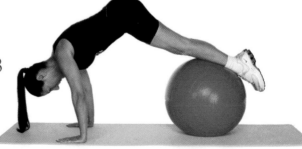

10

A

B

C

D

E

F

G

H

I

K

Index